Understanding Addiction

An LDS Perspective

AF677418

Understanding Addiction

An LDS Perspective

DR. REID WAYNE LOFGRAN

DAY agency

Understanding Addiction
An LDS Perspective
Text Copyright © 2017 by Reid Wayne Lofgran

All rights reserved. No part of this publication may be reproduced, distributed, or transmitted in any form or by any means, including photocopying, recording, or other electronic or mechanical methods, without the prior written permission of the publisher or author, except in the case of brief quotations embodied in critical reviews and certain other noncommercial uses permitted by copyright law. For permission requests, contact the publisher through the website below.

Day Agency
South Jordan, UT 84009
www.dayagency.com

Cover Design and Interior layout: Francine Platt, Eden Graphics, Inc.
Cover image used under license from istockphoto.com
Digital formatting: Dayna Linton, Day Agency

Library of Congress: Pending

ISBN 978-0-9993430-0-5 (Paperback)
ISBN 978-0-9993430-2-9 (Hardback)
ISBN 978-0-9993430-1-2 (eBook)

1. Main Category Non-Fiction—Self-Help
2. Sub Category Non-Fiction— Substance Abuse & Addictions/General
3. Main Category Non-Fiction—Medical
4. Sub Category Non-Fiction—Drug Guides

First Edition
10 9 8 7 6 5 4 3 2 1
Printed in the United States of America

Acknowledgments

Thank you to all those who have helped me with this book:

To my sweet wife for always supporting me, loving me, and being my greatest cheerleader.

To my dear mother, who taught me, and has always believed in me.

To Dr. Douglas O. Smith for starting me on this road.

To my children, (Paul, Tyler, Sami, Zach, Emily, and Kaylee) for bringing such joy to my life.

To Jessica who believed in this project, and put many years into it.

To Richard and Diane who showed me the path.

To Dayna, Fran, and Jenni who guided and helped me along that path.

Dr. Lofgran has written this book to help those who are struggling with addiction, or those who have loved ones struggling with addiction. He has been able to take complex medical terms and neuropsychology and explain them in a way that everyone will understand and be able to apply within their own circumstances, along with the unique addition of gospel principles that will help to heal the ailing spirit.

I have known Dr. Lofgran personally for over 23 years. He is a man of great integrity and faith. He has over 16 years of experience treating those suffering from addiction. He is a former bishop himself which gives him additional insight into healing the spirit as well as the body. I found his application of the atonement and gospel principles to addiction recovery insightful and revolutionary.

His compassionate understanding for the behavioral complexity of chemical dependency will help the reader comprehend, sympathize and even empathize with those suffering from addiction and more fully understand the daunting world and challenges they face. He uses real world examples form his experience working with patients ensnared in the grasp of addiction.

By understanding the biology of addiction through the use of this book, church leaders will be better equipped in helping their youth and adult members avoid the lure of recreational drug use. Furthermore, it will prepare them to adequately respond and provide counsel when confronted with someone who has fallen into addiction. As a practicing family physician and former bishop I can see that this book would be a good resource to help bishops and other church leaders guide them in helping those in their stewardship.

– Dr. Kelly Amann
Family Medicine Physician

Contents

Contents

Section 4: Appendix

Preface

"And we talk of Christ, we rejoice in Christ, we preach of Christ,... that our children may know to what source they may look for a remission of their sins."

2 Nephi 25:26 [1]

As I entered The Walker Center (a 28-day residential addiction treatment facility), I realized the electricity had gone out. I made my way through the dark hallway to the medical office, which I usually used to admit patients to the center. As I put the key in the lock I knew the office would be black and the computer useless. Grabbing the new patient's chart, I met her in the hall.

The patient, a young woman in her early twenties whom I shall call Katrina, was thin to the point of appearing frail. Her long black hair bordered a face wet with tears and strained with the pain of withdrawal. She followed obediently, a degree of fear and anxiety filling her reddened eyes.

We located a windowed room, the light soft but adequate in the fading evening. I invited Katrina to sit, and I sat across the table from her. Without a computer to steal my focus, I became more attentive to her and the task of documenting her disease state. Perhaps that shift is what led to my change in perspective. I questioned her as usual, assessing her drug use to determine the degree of discomfort she would experience as she withdrew from the pain pills she had been abusing. I listened as she told of her parents, who had used drugs while she was a child, how she had stayed sober until her late teens, but her resolve collapsed as life stressors overwhelmed her. She experimented, and what she had perceived as relatively harmless use rapidly consumed her, turning into a deadly pattern of huge doses of IV-injected morphine and other opiates. She cried, in physical and emotional pain, hoping for help, fearing there would be none.

When we finished the interview and the examination, I asked Katrina if she had any questions or concerns, as I usually do. She shook her head, but whispered through a resurgence of tears, "You have all been so kind to me. I thought everyone would be really mean to me and treat me like I am an idiot for doing all the stupid things that got me here." In that moment, something inside me wanted me to help Katrina understand who she is, in God's eyes. Tears came into my eyes as I tried to explain how important it was that she had chosen to get help. She had come to the right place. Despite the difficulties of withdrawal, the risk of relapse, the drug dealers who would prey upon her weak moments, and the stresses of life that would come, she could always get help. I wanted to give her hope in the path she had decided to take.

That night I lay in bed thinking about her words and her situation. Katrina should be living a life of happiness, with her life fully before her. She was in her prime, dark-haired and beautiful, a precious daughter of God in deep trouble. Even though she did not have the gospel in her life, she was still a child of God, with divine potential. I saw myself in her place, with the Savior inviting me to sit and share my trials, sorrows, and failings. I thought how I might expect to be treated like a fool, one who has been given so much, but fallen, impure and unclean, unworthy to be in the presence of the Lord. Yet, I was blessed to know the Lord would not only express His love for me, but also show me how His great plan could heal me. I would feel the gift of His love and find hope in repentance despite my failings. Nothing I could do on my own would return me to the Father's presence. Only accepting the Savior's sacrifice would allow me to return to the Father. The Savior would teach me hope, and show me the way back to my Heavenly Father and the blessings He had for my life.

I then realized the flood of empathy I had experienced during my interview with Katrina was a Christlike love for her—an increased understanding of her suffering, and a deep wish that she would stay on the path to healing and come to know God's plan for her life. Though I had known in my mind the Atonement of Christ applied to every person, I had not felt in my heart the burden of it. That each patient, no matter what mistakes they had made, and despite their feelings of hopelessness and unworthiness, deserved to know the true love of the Savior. A renewed desire to help those trapped in addiction change their lives filled me. Such is the purpose of this book.

The need for this book came to me in 2004 as I sat in a Mexican restaurant in San Diego having dinner with my wife. At the time, I was attending a conference about treating addictions while working to become certified by the American Society of Addiction Medicine as an addictionologist (a physician who specializes in addiction treatment). In my studies, I saw how the science of addiction confirmed the teachings of the Gospel, and I shared this budding field of knowledge with my wife while we waited for our dinner.

Two months prior to this, I had been set apart as a bishop. We were expecting our fifth child in one month and I had only been in medical practice for three years in Gooding, Idaho. Previous to that, we had spent five years training in and around Detroit, Michigan. There we saw up close the world of gangs, violence, drugs, and the general societal loss of morals in which our children would be raised. It greatly concerned us, as I am sure it would any parent. One story hit hard: two girls who had been at a party ended up in an ICU and one of them eventually died. Investigations revealed that GHB (gamma-hydroxy-butyrate) had been added to their drinks. GHB is known as a "date-rape drug," and is generally used to induce a state of emotional susceptibility to suggestion, along with causing amnesia of those events. Sexual predation was likely the intent of the person who spiked their drinks that night. Tragically, a toxic dose had been given, and one of the victims died.

We saw many more tragedies resulting from a society becoming ever more engulfed in the world of drugs and addiction—murders, suicides, increasing crime, and a marijuana leaf inserted into a hamburger at the McDonald's drive-through. A good friend, whose job was as an undercover cop stationed within the drug culture, told us of many such problems. We hoped they were unique to Detroit. But sadly, we have since discovered these dangers are just as much a threat in any town anywhere in America and the world, including our own hometowns.

After Detroit, little of what I encountered as a bishop shocked or surprised me. My years spent working with drug and alcohol addicted patients had convinced me of the real dangers lurking in wait for us and our children. I had heard and seen more tragedy and travail in those eight years than I would previously have imagined possible. Additionally, over the next five years of being a bishop, I realized that through those experiences I had been prepared to understand even more about the trials which members of my ward would face, and I often found myself drawing from my experiences in medicine and in addiction treatment to help those whom I served.

"In 2014, 47,055 deaths involved drug poisoning . . . In 2014, 40% of drug-poisoning deaths involved opioid analgesics (18,893 deaths)."[2]

That evening at the Mexican restaurant while attending the addiction conference in San Diego, my wife (a registered nurse) also expressed her excitement at the progress of medical science in understanding addiction, and with great foresight predicted how that knowledge would help me be a better bishop and help us be better parents. Then she asked how we could help other bishops learn some of these ideas and principles to help those who they served, and we discussed the priceless teachings in the Word of Wisdom. Our conversation and her questions motivated me. I saw how inadequate I would have felt in helping others without having gained my knowledge about addiction and its ravaging effect on the lives of those who fall into its trap. Also, the need for dispelling the misconceptions surrounding the process and the disease of addiction is great, and one of the biggest challenges we face in helping those in need.

"Nearly 88,000 people (approximately 62,000 men and 26,000 women) die from alcohol-related causes annually, making alcohol the fourth leading preventable cause of death in the United States."[3]

How could a 'farmer' bishop, an 'engineer' bishop, a 'school teacher' bishop, or an 'accountant' bishop gain access to information about the many addiction issues plaguing church members in this day? Would they know the street names for drugs? Would they recognize paraphernalia or the drug itself? Would they understand the effects on the body, and how to recognize either intoxication or withdrawal? When youth begin to struggle and slip away, would the parents or leaders even consider addiction as a contributing

The 4 leading causes of death in the United States in 2013 were:

1. Diseases of heart (heart disease)
2. Malignant neoplasms (cancer)
3. Chronic lower respiratory diseases
4. **Accidents (unintentional injuries)**
5. Cerebrovascular disease (strokes)

In 2012 Accidents surpassed strokes in leading causes of death.[4]

Unintentional poisoning deaths (primarily drug overdoses) surpassed motor vehicle accidents as the leading cause of deaths from accidents.

All unintentional injury deaths **(Accidents)**

- Number of deaths: 130,557
- Cause of death rank: 4

Unintentional fall deaths

- Number of deaths: 30,208

Motor vehicle traffic deaths

- Number of deaths: 33,804

Unintentional poisoning deaths (mostly drug overdoses)

- **Number of deaths: 38,851** [5]

factor? And if they had the insight to think of it, would they know how to help? When someone reported a problem with pornography would the bishop simply say, 'just stop doing it'? How could a bishop help someone struggling with an addiction find the right treatments?

There may have been a day in which we did not have to know those things, but that is no longer the case. These problems are everywhere. When I tell people I work with addiction, the conversation often turns to stories of family or friends or acquaintances that are struggling with addiction, have undergone treatment, or overdosed on drugs. Drug addiction is becoming a pervasive problem affecting all of us, and is severely taxing America and the world.

Unfortunately for all of us, we no longer live in a world in which we can stand back and say, "Surely so-and-so could not be using heroine (... or looking at pornography, ... or sexually active, ... or using marijuana, ... or gambling away their living, etc,)." We should consider addiction as a possible cause for those who are struggling spiritually. We must even keep our eyes open for these problems amongst those who appear to have no such trials, for every day we are surrounded by groups of people we know as "functional alcoholics", or "functional addicts", and many who are involved in sins which are devastating to them spiritually, but which we may not recognize. Often it takes the spirit of discernment to perceive such problems, but the more we learn for ourselves, the more the Spirit can use our knowledge to guide us. As I reflected upon this knowledge, I wanted to develop a tool that could help other bishops understand addiction.

My wife and I then considered the need beyond that of bishops. How could parents, youth leaders, teachers, principals, and youth themselves ever understand these things well enough to recognize a problem? How could any of them help those struggling with addictions to find adequate help without knowing the resources available in the field of addiction treatment? It occurred to us how important it is for leaders, parents, and youth to have access to answers and to understand basic concepts of addiction, and how it relates to drugs, pornography, eating disorders, gambling, computer gaming, and other addictions. We wanted to be able to dispense general information that explains these destructive habitual behaviors.

"More than 10 percent of U.S. children live with a parent with alcohol problems, according to a 2012 study." [6]

Amazingly, even though we see how dangerous these things are, these vices seem to hold a fascination for our youth (and even many of our adults). Often, we watch as heartbroken witnesses while people's lives are destroyed by these addictions, which are nothing more than the crafts of Satan. Although my wife and I did not consider ourselves more experienced in the tragedies of these traps, or more knowledgeable than everyone else, we were sure that we had something to offer, if only in raising a voice of warning. We were certain not everyone had lived several years in Detroit and seen the inner workings of such cities, with its drugs, immorality, and violence, as well as the loss of the sacredness of family so rampant everywhere in our world. Through many experiences, including our full-time missions, we had gained a firsthand perspective of the terrible consequences of such lifestyles and the resulting brokenness in so many people's lives.

We were sure most people, especially the youth, had no comprehension of the devastating power of these terribly destructive tools wielded so skillfully by Satan. If they did have any real knowledge or understanding of these things, then why would they ever choose to experiment with them? We concluded the only reason someone would ever choose to participate in behaviors that would bring about such certain spiritual death (and possibly physical death) was they were ignorant

Drug-poisoning and opioid-analgesic poisoning death rates: United States, 2000–2014

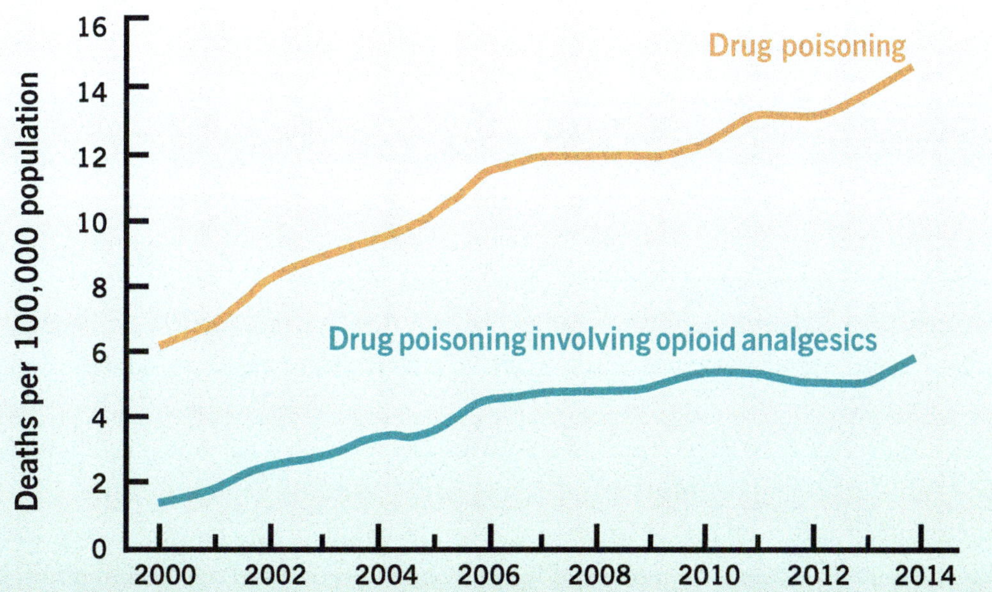

SOURCE: CDC/NCHS, National Vital Statistics System, 2000–2014

[7] (*opioid analgesics = pain medications, narcotics)

of the power of the vices with which they tampered. We were sure few people were truly foolish enough to put their hand in a trap that would not just cut off their hand, but drag them into it entirely, to their utmost destruction. One of the most frequent laments I hear goes something like this: "I had no idea when I started using drugs how terrible this would be. I cannot escape. I wish someone would have helped me understand. If only I could warn others of how horrible this is."

There, in that Mexican restaurant in 2004, we reflected upon our visit the day before to the beautiful San Diego Temple, only a few blocks away. We were struck by the inestimable value of the teachings of the Gospel of Jesus Christ. We discussed the priceless counsel given in the Word of Wisdom, and we reflected upon the divine warnings all of us have had, through scriptures and modern day revelation, to help us avoid the pitfalls Satan has put in our way.

At that moment we considered how so many of our society's problems come about because of our lack of understanding, and because of our naivety as to the extreme danger of the tools and tricks which Satan employs. Satan makes his lures appear so very enticing, and seemingly much more attractive than the gifts and blessings of the Spirit. Yet if only we could see the sorrow and pain of Satan's plan, matched against the joy and peace of the plan of our God, we would never dare to so much as look at Satan's enticements, much less dabble in them.

As Alma expressed in the Book of Mormon, my heart sank at my own incapacity to raise a voice to adequately warn my brothers and sisters of the devastation awaiting anyone who disregards the Lord's counsel concerning these dangers. Yet my heart leapt at the hope that my voice of warning could be heard. If even a few tragedies could be prevented, if even one person could be saved from losing their spiritual identity (since addictive behavior results in the loss of agency) it would be worth the writing of this book. Unlike Alma, who desired to cry forth as with the voice of an angel to all the earth to be heard, we now live in a world capable of instantly sharing knowledge and experience, unprecedented in any previous generation upon this earth.

Through this book, I hope to provide tools to those who are struggling with addiction, or to those that are trying to help someone who is addicted. Most importantly, I want to explain, using ancient and modern revelation, how the Atonement of Jesus Christ does apply to all, even those who feel they are hopelessly trapped by the chains of the Adversary.

I sincerely believe that through faith and prayer and the application of the Atonement of Jesus Christ, all of us can overcome whatever sins beset us, even the most enslaving addictions. However, sometimes we know what we must do, but we lack the knowledge of how to do it, and our pathway is not clear. I pray this book can be part of the answer to someone's personal need, who is seeking the Lord's guidance in finding the path to healing, both physically and spiritually.

Understanding addiction is very important. Even individuals who become dependent on prescribed medications for legitimate uses need to know how to avoid the trap of addiction. Learning which drugs are dangerous and why they are dangerous may help people choose not to use them. Knowing the names, the paraphernalia, and the effects of drugs can help parents or leaders detect problems early. Knowledge can make us free.

To help in this process of learning, this book is designed as follows:

- Chapters 1–14 explain the science and process of addiction, with application to the gospel of Jesus Christ.
- Appendices A–K explain each class of drug, with examples, street names, effects, and other information that will help identify and avoid the most common addictive substances, along with explanations of methods to treat addictions.

SECTION 1

Addiction in Our Lives

CHAPTER 1

Stereotypes

"All I needed was to get sober. I can take care of the rest on my own."

ANONYMOUS ADDICT

The phone rang just after midnight, and I quickly lifted the receiver, hoping my wife could go back to sleep easily. Speaking softly, I answered, seeing the name of the local hospital on the display screen. The physician assistant covering the emergency room greeted me and began telling me about the patient he was now evaluating. The patient was an alcoholic who regularly showed up in the emergency room after he became too drunk to function, or when he became too sick from not having any alcohol. He was very sick right now, and expressed a desire to become sober.

With some degree of skepticism, we decided to admit the patient to the hospital. We would treat him with medications to keep him safe during his detoxification, to prevent seizures or delirium tremens and would request the help of our social worker in finding the patient a treatment program. I went back to sleep.

The next morning, when I saw the patient at the hospital, he expressed gratefulness. The medication had him feeling better. However, discussions with the patient regarding addiction treatment only raised rebuttals about having no time and no money for treatment. He believed, now that he felt better, he could handle recovery all by himself. On the second day, the patient left AMA (against medical advice), even before completely finishing the detoxification process.

Unfortunately, unless a patient has committed to a treatment plan and arranged to spend time at a treatment facility, I have rarely experienced a different outcome when admitting a patient to the hospital for acute drug or alcohol detoxification. As soon as the patient feels better, or feels safe, they leave the hospital and return to their drug of choice. Such behavior has led to a resentment and a pervasive negative attitude among health care providers, and more broadly, among society in general. Addicts and alcoholics often seem a hopeless and unworthy cause.

Addiction is a problem with an extensive history and with complex social implications which are burdened by a host of stereotypical features. Talking of "addicts" conjures up many visions in our minds. These may include the stereotypical homeless alcoholic, the heroin user, the Marlboro man, the reefer addict, the drug dealer, the gangster, etc.

Because of the many misunderstandings about addiction and "addicts," I was hesitant to use the label "addict" in this book for fear the reader would conjure up in his or her mind the socially driven stereotypical concepts of an "addict," rather than learning about the disease of addiction. In the end, I decided to use the term "addict" in hopes that while learning the truth about addiction, the reader would overcome this stereotypical thinking. I also decided to use the term "addict" to refer to anyone with any type of addiction, whether it be drugs, alcohol, or behaviors, as the science is bearing out the reality that the process of addiction is similar in each type.

Often, because of the stereotypes we face in our society's portrayal of addiction, we consider the addict to be someone filthy or with whom we have nothing in common. However, none of us are too far removed from these dangers. Yet, we recklessly label people as addicts, whether they fit any formal definition or not. Perhaps being mortal, and therefore being fallen men and women, none of us are too far removed from the world of addiction. Could it be each one of us has touched the world of addiction ourselves, finding things in our own lives we are unwilling to give up despite the damage they do to us? If we can think of no such physically destructive behaviors, what about our spiritual weaknesses?

We frequently talk about sin, or sinners. The Savior proclaimed, ". . . for I am not come to call the righteous, but sinners to repentance." [1] Are we not all in need of the Atonement of Jesus Christ, and thus all "sinners"? Paul wrote, ". . . that Christ Jesus came into the world to save sinners; of whom I am the chief." [2]

As I learn more about addiction, I see the same concepts underlie the majority of our sins. We refuse to give up that which is destroying us because we love it more than we love righteousness, our agency, our salvation, and our Christ. Until we master the physical body with our spiritual being, we are subject to the desires of that body. In that sense, perhaps, we would all do well to consider the concept of addiction as applying to each of us individually, rather than only to those addicted to drugs, or sex, or gambling, or eating. As Paul confessed to being a "sinner," so should we. Perhaps as we talk about the "addict," we should consider there is a part of the "addict" in every one of us who has not yet become perfected in Christ.

Indeed, the model of addiction has changed over the years from a picture of an individual with a moral character flaw, to a model of disease very similar to other chronic diseases. This is because in chemical addiction we actually see changes in the physiologic function of the body much as we do in other disease processes. These, in turn, overwhelm and control our spiritual being, and our soul becomes lost and fallen. We also know there are significant and powerful genetic influences associated with addiction that help determine if each person will be more physically susceptible to certain habits. Moreover, we know environmental stressors (such as a disrupted home life or childhood abuse) predispose individuals to behaviors which can lead to addictions.

In calling addiction a disease, I do not suggest there is no responsibility for personal choices and actions. If that were the case, then such warnings as those given in The Word of Wisdom would be pointless. As with everything else in this life, we have our agency. Certainly, a poor decision to partake of an addictive substance or participate in an addictive behavior is inevitably what leads one into an addiction. This could also be said of poor dietary decisions in the disease of diabetes, or the growing crisis of obesity in America, and the decision to participate in any spiritually destructive activity in our life. Any activity that takes away our agency (spiritually, emotionally, physically) should be viewed as another tool of Satan.

All too often, people become enslaved by the tools of Satan, against which the Lord has warned us. Then Satan leaves us to rot. As we are taught in Alma, "And thus we see that the devil will not support his children at the last day, but doth speedily drag them down to hell." (Book of Mormon | Alma 30:60). Satan is a cruel task master. He binds us to his ways, enslaves us, and then leaves us lost in the mess. Satan's intent is to destroy us, and leave us as miserable as he is, for eternity. No one should ever be fooled that Satan's long-term plan has anything to do with our happiness, ease, or comfort.

Not long ago, I walked into The Walker Center to admit a patient, and saw a staff member who appeared distressed. I asked her how she was doing. She waved me over, clearly disturbed. She showed me a letter with a picture attached. It was the picture of a young woman who had been through the program approximately six months before. The letter was from the girl's mother who had written to tell us her daughter had overdosed on heroin and died. While in the center, this young woman had done well. She had felt hope, and believed she could overcome the addiction. She had a loving family. She had the church in her life. Once she went home, the pull of the addiction had hold of her, and within a month she had died from an overdose. Such is the story of thousands of people.

Satan did not care about this young woman's well-being. Satan only sought the destruction of a beautiful young daughter of God, to stop all the good she could have done in her life and in the lives of others for generations to come. This is true for any sin in which we become entangled. Satan wants to destroy the valiant children that God has sent to do His work. Despite the apparent allures of a particular lifestyle, the initial euphoria of drug use, the power or wealth or pleasure offered with unrighteous living, the excitement of premarital or extramarital sexual relationships, ultimately the purpose behind all of it is to destroy a child of God who, in truth, has infinite potential.

Any who have been in the bondage of addiction will testify of the terrible power it has over them and of the horrors it brings to their life. Interestingly, those who are in recovery are often the most passionate in helping others who are addicted to understand addiction, along with learning that there truly is a hope of recovery. Perhaps this is because they have been there themselves and understand how terrible it can be, and how it can completely ruin the lives of the addict and those around them. Perhaps recovering addicts and alcoholics have a special opportunity to help those afflicted with the disease, having been there themselves.

However, I believe anyone has the capacity to understand and help fight addiction if they truly understand the love of Christ and the power of His atoning sacrifice. Anyone who has ever repented of a serious sin and felt the peace of forgiveness or felt the spirit of rejoicing in helping others come unto Christ will understand the gift of joy bestowed by the Holy Ghost upon all who choose to follow the Savior. Thus, all people have the capacity to understand addiction, help others escape its chains, and then rejoice in the process of healing.

We all have the opportunity and capacity to help those around us if we take the time and effort to try to understand this disease. These individuals can change. If given the opportunity, these individuals can remove the burden of addiction from their lives, and ultimately receive the same eternal opportunities as those who do not suffer with addictions.

In the world of addiction, it is common to talk about "recovery" rather than being "cured" of addiction. Those who are clean from their addiction are referred to as "recovering." I wholeheartedly embrace this concept. I would note, however, that although we say there is no "cure," and "once an addict always an addict," there is one road to true and complete healing: through Christ, and only through Christ.

CHAPTER 2

Addiction and the Atonement of Christ

"Walking with the Savior in priesthood service will change the way you look at others. He will teach you to see them through His eyes, which means seeing past an outward appearance and into the heart."

President Henry B. Eyring [1]

Early in my career, I admitted a patient to The Walker Center for treatment of opiate addiction. This man, whom I shall call John, was severely discouraged. His story was a story which any of us could experience if we are not watchful and careful. He had been happy, living a good life, with a happy family. He held a position of leadership in his ward for years. John lived his covenants, and was a member in good standing. Then he had a surgery, and was given narcotics for the pain.

"In 2014, an estimated 27.0 million Americans aged 12 or older were current (past month) illicit drug users, meaning that they had used an illicit drug during the month prior to the survey interview." [2]

The time came when John's pain should have been gone, but he did not feel well without the medicine. He still hurt, but looking back, he could not really say that his pain was from the surgery. John continued to get prescriptions from his physician for the pain, even though he was not sure where the pain came from. Every time he tried to stop taking the pain pills, he suffered. Trying to stop the medicine resulted in getting sick to his stomach, cramping in his bowels, hurting all over, and becoming anxious. He would sweat, and his skin would crawl. He could not sleep. He had no idea how to get better, but he did know the pills controlled his symptoms. What he did not understand at the time was that he was experiencing classic opiate withdrawal symptoms.

John explained that after he had been on the pain pills for quite a long time the doctor told him he would no longer prescribe the pain medicines. John began visiting friends and while using their bathrooms he would rifle through their medicine cabinets in search of pain pills. He began pocketing money that he found sitting around on counters and even looking in purses and in drawers to find money because he discovered he could purchase pills online. Then he discovered many other sources of pain pills. He even found people in his community who were willing to sell their pain pills for cash.

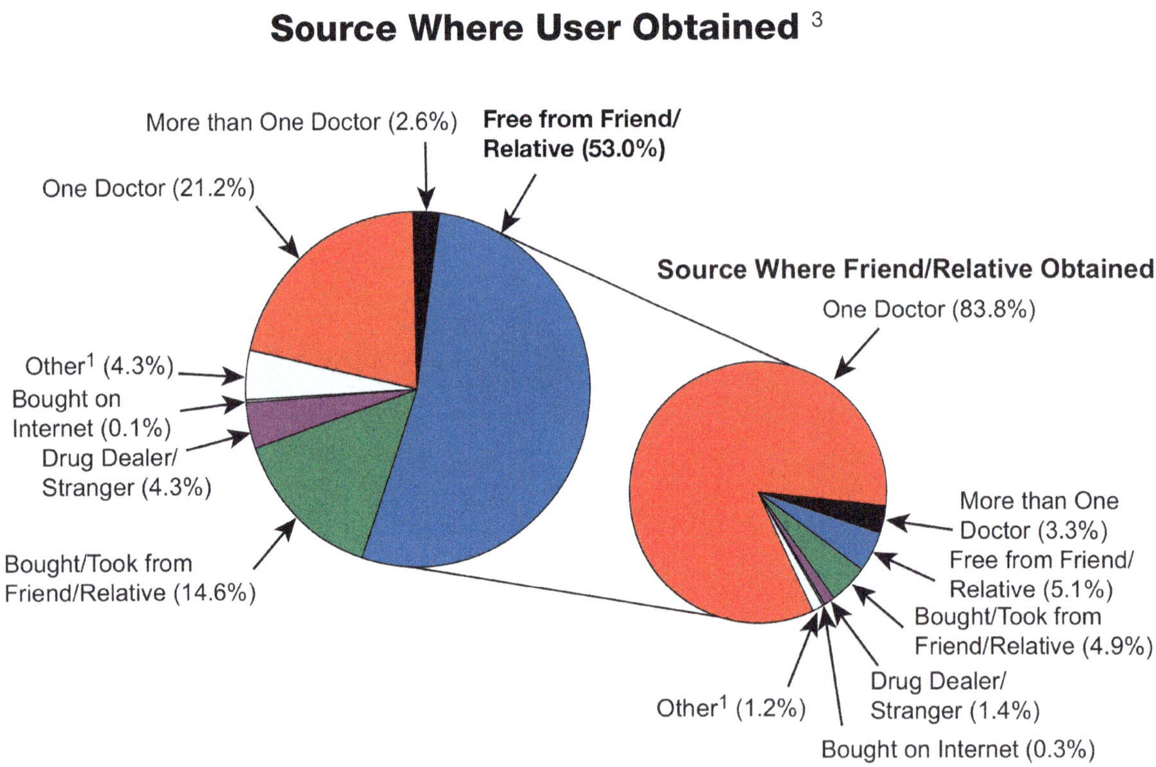

Eventually, John came to a horrifying realization: in order to get more pain pills he did things completely against his beliefs and contrary to the actions of the man he had been his whole life. He had resorted to stealing, lying, and cheating to feed his addiction and he knew he needed help. Despite the embarrassment and humiliation of revealing his actions to his wife and his church leaders, John did seek help. He finally realized the moment he began using the drugs for a different reason than the surgical pain, he could not simply stop on his own. John discovered that though we all have agency, he had given up some of his capacity to choose and act for himself, and was now in the chains and bondage of sin and addiction.

From the very beginning, Satan has desired to take away our agency. The conflict during our pre-mortal life which we often call "the war in heaven" was about Satan wishing to take away our agency, which has been granted unto us by a loving Father in Heaven. One of the fascinating things about this is that Satan could not take away our agency without us exercising that very agency which he sought to take from us. We have to choose to follow him.

Since his first attempt to sabotage our progress, Satan has not changed his plan or purpose. He still desires to take away our agency. We still have the capacity to use that agency to thwart Satan's attacks upon us. However, he frequently changes his tactics and weapons. Though addictions have been around for most of recorded history, I believe the increase in the flow of knowledge and advanced technology has made addictive substances and behaviors more readily available, and much more dangerous. Additionally, Satan, the master of lies, is becoming expert at convincing us these things are really not so dangerous as many would have us believe.

Another tool of Satan critical to understanding in regards to addiction is that of despair and hopelessness. Being overwhelmed and defeated by the stereotype of addiction, and by our failures is one of Satan's greatest ruses. If he can make us believe we are beyond help, or we are not good enough to be loved by God then Satan wins. Satan wants us to believe there is no way out. He wants us to believe no one can ever again love us, or accept us, and we are forever outcasts. This is particularly true within a person's religious community. It is far too easy to believe we cannot come back, especially in the eyes of the people who knew us as an addict. It is also far too easy for Satan to convince us God cannot love us after the terrible things we have done. These are ideas created and perpetuated by Satan.

The beauty of the Gospel message is that through the Atonement of Jesus Christ everyone can be forgiven and partake of the Savior's gift to us, which he paid in Gethsemane. The Savior already paid the price for all of our sins. We only need to accept and apply the principles of faith and repentance, and honor our baptismal covenants.

When Joseph Smith was in the Liberty Jail, he set forth the duty of the Saints in listing their losses and persecutions for the sake of publishing to all the world and the government the wrongs done against the Saints. This was in part to show the craftiness of Satan and his servants, and also to warn those who live in ignorance of the means by which Satan ensnares men and women to evil acts. Verses 13–15 of Doctrine and Covenants Section 123 explain our duty to help those around us, to dispel the lies and myths of Satan, and bring light and knowledge to view. I feel strongly these verses still apply to us today, to any person who has knowledge and can share it for the sake of those around us who are not aware of the lurking dangers waiting to destroy us:

> 13 Therefore, that we should waste and wear out our lives in bringing to light all the hidden things of darkness, wherein we know them; and they are truly manifest from heaven—
>
> 14 These should then be attended to with great earnestness.
>
> 15 Let no man count them as small things; for there is much which lieth in futurity, pertaining to the saints, which depends upon these things. [4]

The mode of persecutions has changed, but Satan is no less vigilant now than he was then. His purpose is to enslave us, and to take away our agency. Few men are willing to simply hand him their agency and become enslaved to him, or to anyone else. We know this because we are all here, having once already made the decision, during our pre-mortal lives, to follow the Savior in sustaining the plan of our Heavenly Father. Satan knows this, and knows there is a more successful way. He tricks us into giving away our ability to act as our own agents in choosing to follow Christ. Satan knows if he can entice us into even one little act of indiscretion that has the potential to addict us, he may then hold the victory over us. Yes—even after just one try!

Any who have seen the evils thrust upon our society by addictions should well understand verse 10 from Doctrine and Covenants Section 123 in the context of our modern society: "Which dark and blackening deeds are enough to make hell itself shudder, and to stand aghast and pale, and the hands of the very devil to tremble and palsy."

Who, having seen the stories of the drug lords, the murders, the victims of destroyed families, lost and abused and exploited children, could doubt the evil surrounding addictions? Who, having seen a baby deformed and debilitated by maternal alcohol consumption during pregnancy, or a newborn withdrawing from opiates following delivery could ever believe that Satan has anything good to offer? Who could watch a previously faithful Latter-day Saint as their life spirals into the loss of job, family, and home, and still doubt that addiction is one of those horrible tools which Satan uses to enslave us?

Past-Month Illicit Drug Use Among Adults Ages 50 to 64 [5]

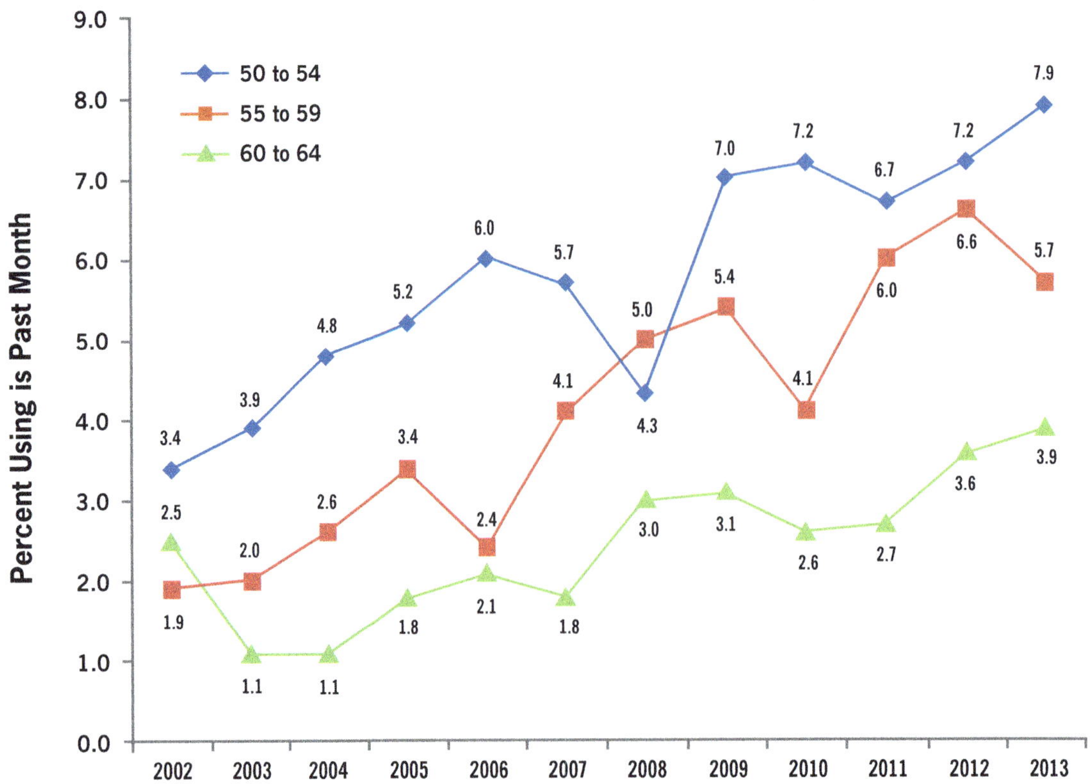

The call to raise the voice of warning is a call which should be given "with great earnestness." As verse 15 concludes, "Let no man count them as small things, for there is much which lieth in futurity. . . ." The Lord was aware of the dangers of our day. He has warned us, given us scriptures, prophets, church leaders, and parents to help us. However, he has also told us that we should "waste and wear out our lives in bringing to light all the hidden things of darkness," and that "these should then be attended to with great earnestness." As much as is possible, I would like to bring to light hidden things relating to addiction.

I see the tragedy of addiction. Every day. I battle alongside those who struggle with their addictions. I offer help, instruction, and resources. However, some will not make use of the greatest healing tool available to them: the Atonement of Jesus Christ. The Atonement of Jesus Christ is the only way by which any of us can be completely healed. Those who do not have faith in Christ, who do not believe they need to apply a spiritual healing into the process of overcoming their addiction, will never find true and complete healing. They may indeed stop their addictive behavior, or abstain from their substance of choice, but they will never truly find the healing which will make them whole.

To invite Christ into our lives, and to apply His atonement through repentance, baptism (and renewing our covenants through the sacrament), being worthy of the companionship of the Holy Ghost, and enduring to the end through making and keeping the covenants of the Holy Temple of God, is the only path to true healing.

This requires us to have the faith to believe, to apply, and then to learn that healing really can happen. To truly believe Christ can heal all wounds and erase all sin is key. To accept that Christ has "descended below them all," and passed beyond all that we may ever suffer, so we know he can understand everything through which we ourselves must pass, helps us develop the faith to be healed. To accept we can become pure and white, despite what we have done, is to know we can overcome all sin. There are no gimmicks, and there is no instant restoration. There are no therapists or practitioners of any form or method of healing who can provide the healing that must occur. They can only offer tools to comfort and stabilize while helping the seeker to understand, accept, and apply the healing of the Atonement of Jesus Christ.

Once one has the faith to depend on the Savior and accept His atonement, the work can go forward. Yet just as the addiction occurred one step at a time, one day at a time, so comes the healing. There is no quick fix. The work is hard and the road is long. Just as each tiny part of the addiction was added to the soul, each little part must be meticulously removed, piece by piece, until we have eliminated it all, just as we added it all, piece by piece.

To remove this from our souls is essential. We must be cleansed from our sins if we are to return to dwell with God. Once we are so cleansed, great blessings await us. Consider what it means when the Lord says, "[T]hen shall thy confidence wax strong in the presence of God . . . ." [6] What a blessing it would be to know that we can stand before God, confident that having done all, we are worthy to be liberated through the Atonement of Christ, and to be sanctified by the Holy Spirit, to abide His presence in confidence! Through our obedience and faith, and the purifying power of

Christ's atonement, we can seek justification, and eventually be sanctified. This is available to all, not just to those who have always attended church. Not just to those who have never had an addiction. Not just to those who have been in church leadership. Salvation is available to all, through the mercy of our Lord, and through the application of the Atonement of Christ. Though it is not an easy road to follow, it is possible through faith, prayer, and living the covenants of salvation.

How many times have we heard the call from our Savior, just as he proclaimed to the ancient Nephites: "Will ye not now return unto me, and repent of your sins, and be converted, that I may heal you? Yea, verily I say unto you, if ye will come unto me ye shall have eternal life. Behold, mine arm of mercy is extended towards you, and whosoever will come, him will I receive; and blessed are those who come unto me." [7]

In the 2010 October General Conference, Elder M. Russell Ballard spoke on addiction and entitled his talk, "O That Cunning Plan of the Evil One." He began his address with this statement: "There is hope for the addicted, and this hope comes through the Atonement of the Lord Jesus Christ." Elder Ballard explains further; "For those of you who have fallen prey to any kind of addiction, there is hope because God loves all of His children and because the Atonement of the Lord Jesus Christ makes all things possible." He then instructs; "It begins with prayer—sincere, fervent, and constant communication with the Creator of our spirits and bodies, our Heavenly Father. . . . Ask to be filled with the power of Christ's pure love." [8]

We can all rejoice in the knowledge that there is hope, even for those with addictions. The Savior will lift us. He will help us. He will heal us. We simply have to be willing to reach out, take His hand, and follow the path He has set for us.

CHAPTER 3

Appetites and Addictions

"Come unto me, all ye that labour and are heavy laden, and I will give you rest."

Matthew 11:28 [1]

Perhaps to understand the process of addiction we need to first take a step back and see how it applies to every one of us. In the Book of Mormon King Benjamin taught us the following:

> "For the natural man is an enemy to God, and has been from the fall of Adam, and will be, forever and ever, unless he yields to the enticings of the Holy Spirit, and putteth off the natural man and becometh a saint through the atonement of Christ the Lord, and becometh as a child, submissive, meek, humble, patient, full of love, willing to submit to all things which the Lord seeth fit to inflict upon him, even as a child doth submit to his father." [2]

The Natural Man is the exact opposite of the Spiritual Man. Our soul, according to Doctrine and Covenants 88:15, is the combination of our spirit body and our physical body. The carnal, or natural, man is the person who has allowed the appetites of the flesh to overcome their spiritual desires and sensitivities. To become spiritual, then, is exactly the opposite; the spirit must overcome and control the desires and appetites of the physical body. Thus, we understand better Brigham Young's teachings:

> "If the spirit yields to the body, the Devil then has power to overcome the body and spirit of that man, and he loses both." [3]

In his epistle to the Galatians, the apostle Paul also taught this principle as he set forth the "works of the flesh and the fruits of the Spirit." Such characteristics are described in Galatians 5:16–25, and include traits of the flesh and of the spirit. Attributes of those who succumb to the appetites of the physical body include adultery, fornication, uncleanness, lasciviousness, idolatry, witchcraft, hatred, variance, emulations, wrath, strife, seditions, heresies, envyings, murders, drunkenness, revellings, and such. Attributes of the spirit include love, joy, peace, long-suffering, gentleness, goodness, faith, meekness, and temperance. We could add many other characteristics to each of these lists, but those listed certainly provide us with a good idea of the types of qualities applicable to either spiritual or physical application.

Much of the purpose of this life seems to be the need to learn how to control the appetites of this physical body which we have been given. This is a key concept as we address the issue of almost any temptation or difficulty in this life. Examine the appetites listed below, and you will see they, in fact, are simply related to the physical desires of our bodies. Notice also these appetites are generally necessary for the survival of our physical bodies, or to create and sustain posterity, or to have the means by which to do good in this world, but any of them in excess can lead to the addictions, diseases, and ailments we see in our world.

1. Eating and Exercise

Eating is, of course, essential for survival. However, we are also learning eating in excess or in imbalance (eating preferentially foods that are easy to get or more appealing rather than healthy) contributes to most of the major diseases that account for morbidity and mortality in our society: heart disease, cancer, diabetes, hypertension, and many other diseases related to obesity, high cholesterol, etc. Additionally, exercise and weight loss can be very important for our health.

2. Sex and Procreation

Men and women are naturally attracted to one another, and properly so. The first commandment given to Adam and Eve was to multiply and replenish the earth—but given under the sacred covenant of marriage. However, Satan twists it and wants us to believe that sexual desires are to be felt and expressed far beyond their purpose or without the sacred covenants associated with their proper use. This is seen in premarital sex, extramarital sex, sexual abuse, pornography, and other sexual practices now accepted in society but contrary to the commandments. Some of the results of uncontrolled sexual appetites include broken homes and marriages, children born into single parent homes, sexually transmitted diseases, deeply seated emotional pain and psychiatric illnesses, and more.

3. Drugs

Many medications are life-prolonging and even life-saving if used correctly. For example, foxglove can be deadly in its natural form, but when it is purified and the dose is controlled it can be life-saving in the form of digitalis, which helps to keep a damaged heart from beating too fast. Other medications mimic chemicals in our bodies, and can be a great blessing, such as when treating extreme pain. However, if overused such pain medications can lead to terrible addictions. Other drugs such as alcohol, nicotine, and marijuana have found ways into legal acceptance into our society, even while having potentially terrible long-term effects. There are a few chemicals (or drugs) that have never been found to have a physiologic benefit, but they are abused due to the effects they have upon the brain.

4. Entertainment

We have many ways of entertaining ourselves, and always have. We dance and sing, go boating, skiing, backpacking, hunting and enjoy the outdoors in many ways. We watch high school, college, and professional sports. We enjoy orchestras and musicals. We watch movies, play board games and computer games. We shop in many venues, and play games on the internet. These can be done appropriately, but in excess can all be damaging. We are cautioned over and over not to allow any form of entertainment to override our duties and responsibilities such as family, work, and church service. Some of the more recent issues of concern are gambling and online computer gaming. A simple example of how these become a concern is the large number of college students who are failing out of college because they spend so much time in their virtual computer worlds. Another example is the almost complete abandonment of the Sabbath Day for the sake of entertainment and pleasure in our society.

5. Power

Power can be obtained in many ways—through honest work, money, politics, persuasion, religion, etc. Power can be a wonderful tool if it is power obtained by doing good, for the sake of doing good. Yet power for the sake of power becomes extremely dangerous. It is also very tantalizing, and seems to be the focus of much of what motivates the world today and throughout history. If power is sought for the purpose of doing wrong, it will destroy the soul. And even power sought to do good can cause destruction if the means to gain it are not consistent with God's law.

6. Wealth

Wealth (or perhaps the willingness to sacrifice wealth) provides the capacity to help many people and bless the lives of others. It is the sacrifice of wealth that allows temples to be built, missionary work to be done, universities to function, meeting houses to be maintained, relief to be administered to the needy, and humanitarian aid to be sent to areas of disaster. Wealth allows for the improvement of our living conditions. Wealth allows us to improve our health. Wealth allows for invention and distribution of new technologies. Yet if it becomes a means unto itself, it is simply another form of power that can twist and corrupt. The issue is whether the wealth becomes the motivating factor, or is it simply another tool used to do good. Nephi's brother Jacob taught:

> "Think of your brethren like unto yourselves, and be familiar with all and free with your substance, that they may be rich like unto you. But before ye seek for riches, seek ye for the kingdom of God. And after ye have obtained a hope in Christ ye shall obtain riches, if ye seek them; and ye will seek them for the intent to do good—to clothe the naked, and to feed the hungry, and to liberate the captive, and administer relief to the sick and the afflicted." [4]

In and of themselves, none of these things listed above are evil, and it can even be argued they are all essential for our health and well-being. However, we can also see these things can be a foundation upon which Satan can build. If he can convince us to misuse any of these things, we then find ourselves succumbing to the flesh, the "Natural Man."

Talking to his son Corianton, Alma teaches us the following:

> "And now, my son, all men that are in a state of nature, or I would say, in a carnal state, are in the gall of bitterness and in the bonds of iniquity; they are without God in the world, and they have gone contrary to the nature of God; therefore, they are in a state contrary to the nature of happiness." [5]

Therefore, we see that it is impossible to be living in a "state of nature" (or living upon the gratifications of our physical appetites—letting our body make the decisions rather than our spirit) and expect to have God and peace in our lives. Instead, we are in bonds, and without God. Eternal happiness is not found through listening to the appetites of our flesh.

In our current world one of the biggest challenges we face is the "loudness" of everything around us. We raise our children hoping that they will hear the peace and calm of the Still Small Voice. Instead, we find ourselves being swept away by music, movies, amusement parks, video games, and access to nearly everything we could dream of with only the sacrifice of a little cash. Eventually, we find ourselves consumed by the overwhelming press to get more money to entertain ourselves further. Where in this noise do we have a place for the Holy Spirit to reach us?

As we become consumed more and more by the attempts to satisfy our appetites, we have a hard time appreciating the rewards of the Holy Spirit in our lives. We and our children miss the soft voice, the simple peace that is the reward of the Spirit, because of the clamor of our appetites striving to be satisfied within our mortal bodies. The body begins to control us, and instead of becoming Spiritual beings, we become the "Natural Man".

When we look back later in our lives we may see more clearly how rewarding it is to live by the Spirit because we then understand the cost of satisfying those physical appetites. We see the terrible struggles of the addict. We see the pains and sorrow of sin, and the toil of repentance. We see the complications of unhealthy lifestyles as we struggle with diseases we might have avoided. We also see the gradual unraveling of the fabric of our society as more and more people move away from their moral framework and values, forcing society to impose boundaries and limits upon them to prevent chaos and the destruction of that society. Then we see society begin to crumble and cave to pressure from the overwhelming forces of individuals who have chosen to justify their lack of morals. We watch as individual rights and uncontrolled personal preferences without acceptance of consequence unravel the framework of a society built upon God-given freedoms.

In contrast we see how, as King Benjamin declared, when we yield to the enticings of the Holy Spirit and put off the natural man, we then find joy, peace, and happiness. Upon reflection, we will find these to be so much more desirable and delicious than the brief gratification of our physical appetites that then lead us into pain and sorrow. It is, as Lehi said of the fruit of the tree of life, the most desirable above all fruits.

Along with these appetites we often become consumed by the biggest appetite—"ME". Amidst all of these trials and troubles we would all find a greater measure of the Spirit by reaching out to others in service and love. This is, in fact, one of the guiding principles behind the healing of addictions—get out and serve and help others who struggle with the same problem. We find our appetites diminished, our desires for self-satisfaction and gratification much assuaged when we lose ourselves in the service of others. Again, King Benjamin taught;

> "And behold, I tell you these things that ye may learn wisdom; that ye may learn that when ye are in the service of your fellow beings ye are only in the service of your God." [6]

Where would we find greater healing and a greater measure of the Spirit as our companion than by choosing to be in the service of our God?

With an understanding of the basic needs of our body (the Natural Man) as the source of destructive behaviors, perhaps we can now all understand addiction a little better. Perhaps we all have a vice, a little appetite that we have a hard time "giving away". As King Lamoni's father said to Aaron,

> "O God, Aaron hath told me that there is a God; and if there is a God, and if thou art God, wilt thou make thyself known unto me, and I will give away all my sins to know thee . . . ." [7]

We all must be willing to ultimately "give away my [our] sins" in order to know God. We may not see our own faults as being at all related to the actions of an addict. However, whatever appetite of the body we allow to control our decisions will eventually follow the same path as the "addict". It gratifies the physical being using biochemical pathways similar to those in addictions, and leads to the need for repentance. The intensity varies, but the process is the same. How hard is it for us to give up our very favorite food if it is placed in front of us after a long fast Sunday? Do we think to ourselves, 'Oh, just this once won't matter? If I don't eat it now, I will lose that chance.'?

How hard is it to give up the idea that we must have our cable TV or computer games? How hard is it to watch our children cry because they cannot have the toys or the clothes that their friends have, without giving in to them? How hard is it to accept living in a very small house, struggling to buy groceries when the neighbors "have it all", or perhaps even harder to give it up when we have it all, to help the poor neighbor who struggles to keep food on the table? These are all based on our own perception of what we need, and if they are physically-based then they are different from the addict's "needs" only in intensity, yet sometimes not in behavior.

Consider, for the sake of understanding, hunger. Anyone who has fasted understands hunger. When we were children, it seemed nearly impossible for us to go without food for twenty-four hours. As we mature, however, we find that we can overcome the hunger and learn to go twenty-four hours without food, assuming we don't have an illness that prevents us from doing so. But in fasting for 24 hours we have the understanding it will come to an end because we have the means to provide ourselves with food. We hope to get to the point with fasting that we can turn it into a spiritual experience while we learn to overcome a physical appetite. Most of us will never die from fasting for 24 hours. However, we are certainly eager to eat when the time comes, and happily give in to our body's cries for nourishment.

Yet, let us consider what would happen if we were in the wilderness, and had not had any food to eat for 3 days. Then our hunger would begin to consume our thoughts. We would realize that if we do not find food we could die (despite the reality that for most people, they could live for several weeks without food). Our thoughts focus on food. Our behaviors focus on finding food. Our behaviors and attitudes then reflect our concerns about the sustainability of our lives. Most other concerns in our lives become secondary to finding something to eat.

Unfortunately, with some addictions, going without the addicting substance can be life-threatening. Other addictions feel life-threatening. Some patients in withdrawal literally feel like they are going to die. It is easy, then, to see why their lives become consumed in trying to find the next dose of the addictive substance.

To the person afflicted with an addiction, this behavior brought on by an appetite becomes more and more difficult to "give away." They have a harder and harder time recognizing there is any problem other than getting more of the addictive substance, for the sake of survival, real or perceived. They become distracted from the important things in life. They focus only on those things which will make them feel stable. Other issues become less meaningful, relative to what they perceive as their more immediate, life-sustaining needs.

Again, perhaps, we can relate to this in our own lives. How often have we sat in a church meeting, or at a fireside, or listened to conference and heard something, knowing it applied to us, but then quickly convinced ourselves it did not really mean us, or what we are doing doesn't hurt anything, or it's not important right now, or it does not really apply to me – How often do we tell ourselves we can control it?

Any of us who have ever had these feelings can understand a little of the disease of addiction, but with much less intensity in the power and strength of the appetite controlling us. In the end, it comes down to a question of recognizing the disease, or the appetite and its reward, as a problem. Then we have to seek help. Most people cannot do it by themselves.

To help us better understand the disease of addiction, we will next embark on a discussion of what science is learning about addiction.

SECTION 2

THE SCIENCE OF ADDICTION

CHAPTER 4

What is Addiction?

"According to the dictionary, addiction of any kind means to surrender to something, thus relinquishing agency and becoming dependent on some life-destroying substance or behavior."

– M. Russell Ballard [1]

At some point in our lives all of us have known an addict. Often times, however, we associate this only with addiction to drugs and are even confused about the differences between abuse, dependence, tolerance, and addiction. Not only is it difficult to clearly understand what these terms mean and how they differ, but it is also complicated to tell how they apply to the use and abuse of different substances.

Then there is the problem of distinguishing between the individual who seems to abuse drugs of some sort, but remains quite functional, versus the one who becomes extremely intoxicated with only one drink of alcohol. Many people misunderstand which of those individuals is actually at more risk of becoming addicted. To complicate things further, we find that addictive behaviors even stretch into realms we often overlook, such as gambling, eating disorders, sexual addictions, abuse patterns, and more.

Many myths and stereotypes cloud our understanding and our capacity to effectively deal with addictions. We are easily enmeshed into the manipulative behaviors often exhibited by addicts, and soon find ourselves enabling the addiction despite our best efforts to fight against it. As with many things, addiction requires first a basic understanding of the physiology and chemistry of addiction. Then once we understand what it is and how it works, we can learn how to deal with it.

Terminology is a logical and essential place to begin any discussion. There are different definitions in the language of addiction, depending on whether one works in the field of psychiatry, psychology, medicine, counseling, etc. It is important to know that many of the terms and definitions used in medical fields are used to determine billing charges for medical or behavioral services.

Recently, the language used has changed to try and clarify several terms for the sake of insurance billing and treatment classification. The most result publication, the DSM V (Diagnostic and Statistical Manual of Mental Disorders Fifth Edition) describes addiction and abuse as a spectrum of disorders, which are now called "substance use disorders." For example, in the past we might have said alcohol abuse, or alcohol addiction, whereas now these are collectively called alcohol use disorder.

To discuss these issues clearly, it is critical to define these terms of abuse simply. These are simplifications, which I have summarized consistent with concepts found in the American Society of Addiction Medicine's (ASAM's) Textbook, *Principles of Addiction Medicine*, 4th Edition,[2] as well as from addiction journals and lectures.

1. Abuse	Incorrect use of any substance.
2. Dependence	When the lack of the drug or behavior results in withdrawals.
3. Tolerance	The need to increase the dose to achieve the desired effect.
4. Addiction	Repeated behavior that results in damage or loss to oneself and others.
5. Recovery	Process of healing from abuse, dependence, tolerance, or addiction.
6. Denial	Failure or refusal to accept that one has a problem.
7. Abstinence	Staying away from an addictive substance or behavior, or never trying such.
8. Relapse	Slipping back into abuse or addiction.

1. Abuse:

The use of potentially addictive or harmful substances (which could also be related to risky, potentially harmful, or dangerous behaviors) in any inappropriate setting. This could include illegal use of a substance, use of illegal substances, or incorrect use of legal prescriptions. Often abuse has readily-visible adverse effects, but not always. Unfortunately, it often leads to continued use and addiction. Such misuse frequently becomes a legal issue.

- Someone who binges on alcohol on weekends.
- A high school "kegger."
- Under-aged experimentation with any legal controlled or illegal substance, such as alcohol, tobacco, marijuana, pain pills, sedatives, etc.
- Taking a family member's prescription medication, regardless of the reason, when not under the advice and care of a professional who can legally prescribe it.
- A one-time trial of marijuana at a party.
- Excessive or ongoing use of prescription drugs when no longer needed.
- Excessive use of over-the-counter medications to get a "buzz."
- Use of any medications (even over the counter) for a reason other than its indicated use.

2. Physical (or Physiologic) Dependence:

Use of a substance such that the physiology of the body adapts to the substance, thus causing withdrawal symptoms if the substance is abruptly stopped, or cravings for the substance once it is depleted in the body. This does not necessarily imply abuse or addiction, simply that the body has developed a dependence on the substance, and therefore, a need of the substance in order to continue to function normally. Unfortunately, this often leads to abuse or addiction, in hopes of helping the body feel normal, or for an individual to function normally.

- Use of opiates post-surgically for several weeks, and when the medication is stopped, flu-like symptoms develop.
- Irritability or restlessness in the mornings while waiting for the coffee to percolate.
- Irritability and cravings while waiting for the smoking break at work.
- Inability to sleep if a sleeping pill is discontinued.
- Severe constipation after prolonged use of laxatives.

3. Tolerance:

Changes in the body's processes of sensing or metabolizing a substance such that over time the substance has less and less effect, often resulting in a gradual increase in the amount or frequency of use of that substance in order to obtain the desired effect.

- When abusing drugs, addicts have to continue to increase the dose of the drug in order to maintain the desired high.
- In chronic pain treatment, the dose of pain medicine often has to be escalated to maintain adequate pain control.

- The desired effects of controlling sleep and anxiety problems dwindle after extended use of a medication, resulting in ever-increasing doses to produce the desired results.
- Ability to tolerate more and more alcohol in one sitting, with ever-increasing serum alcohol levels, but seemingly less intoxication.

4. Addiction:

A maladaptive pattern of substance use that leads to a combination of effects possibly including tolerance, withdrawals, escalation in doses, unsuccessful attempts at reducing use, and more focus and activities spent on obtaining the substance. However, the most significant indicator of addiction is the repeated and ongoing use of a substance (or persistence of a behavior) despite adverse outcomes to the user and those around them—such as the loss of family, job, home, etc. in exchange for continuation of using the substance. Denial of the problem tends to be a tragically difficult hurdle for those with a true addiction.

- Homelessness, broken families, unemployment.
- Legal problems, incarceration, drug courts.
- The methamphetamine user who is starving to death because their only thought is "Where do I get the next dose?"
- The teenager who leaves family and church and security prematurely because they cannot give up the pain pills or marijuana in the face of the conflict it creates at home and within themselves.
- The mother whose children are taken by the state because she cannot quit using drugs, despite the loss of those to whom she gave life.
- The man whose pornography problem has led to his excommunication and the estrangement of his wife and children.
- The teenage girl who cannot enjoy a healthy relationship after reading too many sexually explicit books, which alter her perceptions of love and romance.
- The struggling Christian who cannot give up that one vice, despite the despair that follows, when the Holy Spirit can no longer abide with that person.

Dependence, tolerance, and abuse can lead to addiction. However, they are often confused with addiction. An individual who has been on pain medications for a chronic pain condition often finds that over time the medications become less effective. That individual may find their dosage increased until they are on a tremendously high dose. This is clearly a tolerance (and likely dependence) to the medicine, but if they have used it according to prescription, then it is neither abuse nor addiction.

In most cases if they stop the medication they will experience withdrawal symptoms, showing that they also have a physical (or physiologic) dependence to the medication. However, if they have never misused or sought to obtain the medications above their prescribed amounts and have complied with the physician's treatment guidelines, then they have never abused the medications. Furthermore, if the use of these medications has not been the cause of losing jobs or breaking up marriages, this may not fit the criteria of addiction. Unfortunately, these individuals still may need to go through detoxification and treatment programs to become free of the substances to which they have become dependent or tolerant.

On the other hand, a person may heavily use alcohol, but under duress confess a desire and willingness to quit. They stop, experiencing only minor withdrawal symptoms, and maintain sobriety for a time, making this appear to be a controllable behavior and thus more of an abuse situation than an addiction. However, this may be followed by a simple indiscretion of one drink and then a relapse into heavy alcohol use, confirming the presence of an addiction and validation to the concept that addicts who discontinue use of their addictive substance are in recovery, not cured.

5. Recovery:

State or condition of abstinence following an addiction or drug dependence. It is common to talk about addiction as incurable. Those who have controlled the addiction are referred to as being in recovery. In most addictions, longer and longer periods of abstinence result in increased ability to abstain from the drugs or behaviors. However, the reality still exists that as little as one single dose of the substance of choice often results in immediate recurrence of the addiction process.

6. Denial:

The state or condition where an individual does not accept that he or she has a problem. They are unwilling or unable to recognize that the source of their pains and sufferings is the addictive substance or behavior. Yet they suffer from the addiction, and those around them see them suffer and often suffer themselves. They may be too ashamed to admit they have a problem, or too proud to accept that they have made a bad choice and are caught up in something beyond their control. They may be in too much despair, and feel there is no hope for them and they can never recover, much less be forgiven. They may love the substance or behavior too much, or be too dependent on it, and feel there is no way they can overcome those powerful physical cravings. They may simply not be capable of feeling the quiet influence of the Holy Spirit, prompting them to change their life. Generally speaking, those caught up in any bad behavior, including addiction, do not excel in rational thinking. Alcohol is one good example. Most individuals who have an alcohol use disorder do not think they have a problem, as shown in the graph on the following page.

Perceived need for treatment among individuals aged 21–64 who meet criteria for alcohol abuse disorder or alcohol dependence disorder and have not received alchohol treatment at a specialty facility* in the past year: 2006–2009

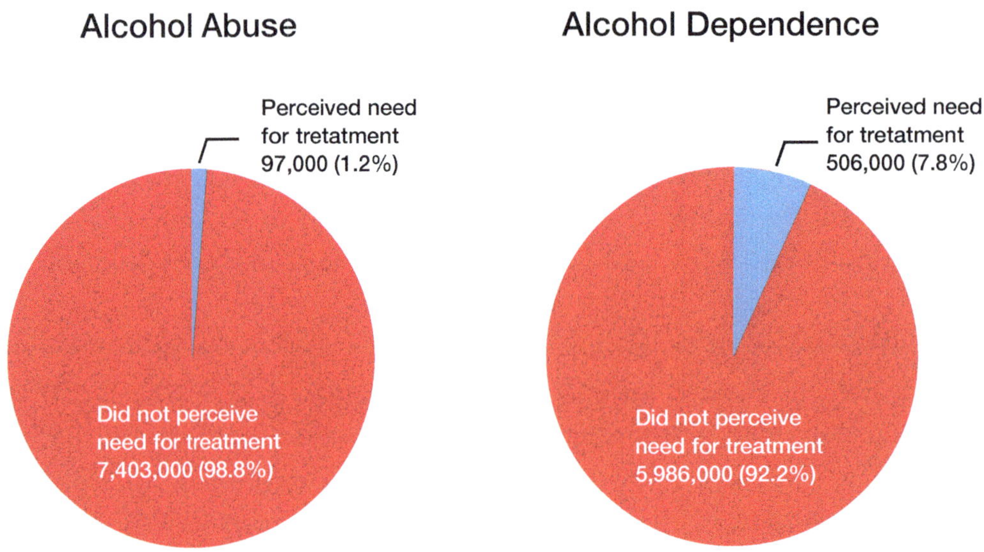

*Received alchohol treatment at at specialty facility refers to treatment received at a hospital (inpatient) rehabilitation facility (inpatient or outpatient) or mental health center in order to reduce or stop alcohol use or for medical problems associated with alcohol use. Specialty alcohol treatment excludes treatment in an emergency room, private doctor's office, self-help group, prison or jail, or hospital as an outpatient.

7. Abstinence:

Never using a substance or participating in a given behavior. This is also used to describe staying away from or being clean from addictive substances. This can apply both to behaviors and substance abuse. Abstinence in its truest form of never indulging in a substance or behavior would, of course, prevent addiction. However, abstinence is often used to describe stopping and then staying away from a substance or behavior once it has become addictive to a person. This is a critical component of recovery.

In our society, abstinence is frequently referenced in connection with avoiding sexual promiscuity or as a means of preventing pregnancy. Abstinence in sexual behaviors, as explained by our church leaders, is described as no sexual relations before marriage. Interestingly, it should be noted many of the same chemical pathways triggered in drug addiction are also triggered by certain behaviors that can be addicting, including sexual behaviors. Abstinence is the only way to truly avoid ever triggering the processes of abuse or addiction with chemicals or behaviors.

8. Relapse:

Falling back into a pattern of abuse or behavior involved in the addiction. Unfortunately, this is one of the defining characteristics of the disease of addiction. While it is obviously the ideal hope that relapse never occurs, those who deal with any person who has an addiction need to understand this is a pattern of behavior typical of the changes that have been rendered by the addiction. Relapse does not mean an individual is hopeless. Relapse does not mean an individual cannot change. In reality, relapse is part of addiction, and is an indicator an individual is truly addicted and needs help to control the addiction.

At one time, I heard an addiction counselor lamenting the poor success of addiction recovery programs, as attested by the rate of relapse. My response to this was that we cannot afford to measure the success of recovery efforts by the percentage of relapse. What is much more telling is whether or not the individual has been given the tools to know where to go for help and realize that they need assistance in that critical moment of relapse. If they return for support and are able to again walk the road to recovery, then theirs is not a failure. It is a temporary setback, during which they hopefully learned a lot about themselves and about the disease of addiction.

Again, as we consider the circumstances of relapse and wonder how an individual could ever go back to that terrible life, we require but a moment of self-reflection. Any of us who condemns the addict for relapse need only find the time in our own life when we chose to again commit a sin (little or big) of which we had once repented. Having done so, we let go of the repentance and forgiveness we had once obtained, and have to start anew the process of seeking a path back from spiritual death. Just as the addict, then, seeks to resume the path of recovery, we too must seek the path of rebirth, through the Atonement of Jesus Christ.

CHAPTER 5

Neurotransmitters What are They?

"In reality, scientific research is an endeavor to ascertain truth."

Howard W. Hunter [1]

For years science has studied and searched to understand what is behind the process of addiction. Now decades of research are available to explain the process of addiction. As we learn more about addiction we are better able to understand the principles taught by Christ and his prophets over the past several Millennia are meant to help us avoid being trapped by the Natural Man. If we have never had a chemical or behavioral addiction then it is very difficult to understand the power of addiction. Looking to science to help explain how addiction works and why it happens is an important part in helping those suffering from this disease.

For most people, it is difficult to understand what it truly is like to be addicted to something. While a number of things can trigger addictive-like responses in the body, only a few of them are strong enough (if processed in a normal way) to lead to addiction. So, what happens for an individual whose response goes beyond this level? A release of chemicals in the brain associated with behaviors necessary to our survival occurs and creates a pathway upon which an addiction can form. One of the most important of these processes is the release of dopamine within the brain.

Dopamine is a neurotransmitter, and is the key neurotransmitter in addictive processes because it is the primary neurotransmitter in the reward system of our brain. It makes us happy. It makes us feel good when we do something like eating food. It is triggered by many behaviors and by many other chemicals and neurotransmitters. It is the final step in our brain telling us it really likes what we just did.

Neurotransmitters such as dopamine are at the heart of addiction. There are certainly many other chemicals and processes which drive behaviors, such as various types of hormones (testosterone, estrogen, and adrenaline, to name a few). However, neurotransmitters seem to be the driving force behind the process of addiction itself. Much research has gone into discovering neurotransmitters and defining their roles in the body. Before we discuss the roles of various neurotransmitters, a short discussion of neuroanatomy is important.

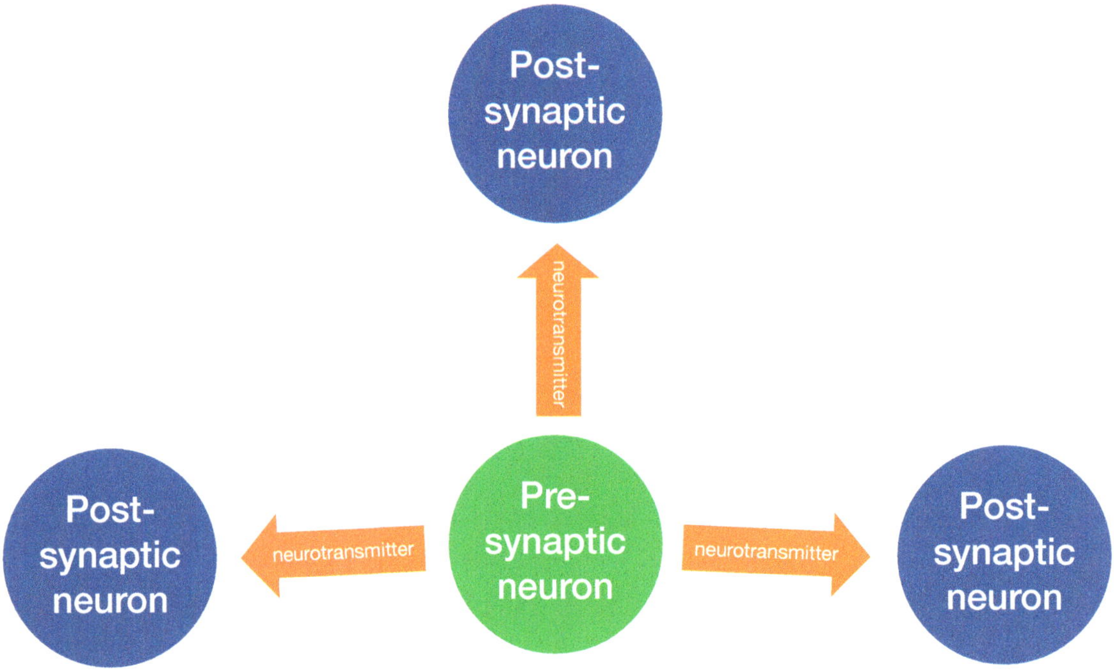

A neurotransmitter is simply the chemical which causes a signal to be sent from one nerve cell (neuron) to another, thus allowing transmissions of messages, and essentially mediating all the functions of the nervous system. There is a space between two nerves that is known as a synapse. A neurotransmitter takes the message from the nerve that originates the signal ("pre-synaptic neuron") across the space to the next nerve ("post-synaptic neuron"). There may be multiple nerves (post-synaptic neurons) which receive the signal.

To simplify, imagine for a moment we are on an aircraft carrier in the middle of the Pacific Ocean. We suspect there is a submarine hunting us, so we need to mobilize a smaller, faster vessel to find and destroy the submarine before it destroys us. We decide to send a signal to a certain destroyer in our fleet, but on the high seas it would be impossible to maneuver the ships close enough to talk to the commander of the destroyer. Instead, we pick up the radio and hail the destroyer captain, using their specific call-name. When the destroyer's captain hears our instructions, he carries out his duties to hunt the enemy submarine.

Think of the aircraft carrier as the first nerve in the sequence, or the "pre-synaptic" neuron. The destroyer is the "post-synaptic" neuron. The distance between our aircraft carrier and the destroyer is the synapse. The radio signal that allows transmission of our orders to the destroyer is the neurotransmitter. Each vessel in the fleet has a predetermined role in the fleet's overall purpose, just as each neuron has a predetermined role in the body. Each radio message has a specific target and will start a defined process, just like each neurotransmitter has a signal it will transmit, and a neuron it will set in action. The key to the integrated function of the fleet is the radio communication between the vessels, just as the key to the integrated function of the body is the host of neurotransmitters between the neurons.

Reward pathways in our brains are, at least in part, controlled by neurotransmitters. Hundreds of neurotransmitters are suspected of being involved, and we are constantly learning of more, while coming to a better understanding of those that have been identified.

One of the most universal and better understood of the neurotransmitters is dopamine. This particular chemical has many functions, but one of them is to stimulate the neurons within the brain leading to rewards for certain behaviors. The reward is so powerful that dopamine is very effective at reinforcing any behavior which leads to a dopamine release. This means when we do something enjoyable (such as eating), dopamine is released, and we feel so good about that activity a wonderful memory is created, and we want to experience it again and again and again. This can apply to almost anything we enjoy. The intensity of the reward will vary greatly with our physiologic response to whatever it is we did. As a general rule, the more we enjoyed it the first time, the more we will want to do it again. Subsequent events that continue to be enjoyable will reinforce our desire to continue to repeat that activity. The more frequently we do them, the more enforcing they are.

A common example of dopamine release is what happens when someone eats chocolate. There are, of course, some people who do not enjoy chocolate. This simply means their brain does not release dopamine when they eat chocolate—they don't like chocolate. However, for most people there is a substantial release of dopamine when they eat chocolate.

We often associate dopamine with drug use and addiction, but we see this same reward system in many other behaviors, such as eating chocolate. Over the years, I have seen how chocolate really can give us a model of behavior reinforced by dopamine release. (If you do not like chocolate, then think about your very favorite food or dessert instead of chocolate). Not only do we experience a dopamine release after eating chocolate, but as we repeat the behavior, our brain begins to anticipate the effects of eating the chocolate. If you are a chocolate lover you will understand that eventually even when we talk about or think about eating chocolate we can remember how good it was, and how much pleasure it brings to us when we eat it. After we have indulged in chocolate multiple times, just the thought of the chocolate will cause a release of dopamine, even before we eat it. This becomes a strong motivation for repeating behaviors. Now we have, in a sense, already had a taste of the chocolate (chemically within our brain), and really want to have it again to get the complete satisfaction.

Having looked at that model as it relates to chocolate, let's consider an addictive substance. Nicotine is one of the most addictive substances because it causes rapid dopamine release and is frequently and rapidly reinforced, as people smoke multiple cigarettes a day. It is typically self-administered, so the dose is solely dependent on whether the smoker is craving it or not. Since the effects wear off quickly it is rapidly repeated. All of these factors contribute to nicotine being so highly addictive.

Let's say that someone named Sam has decided to quit smoking after years of being a smoker. We already know the years of smoking have caused Sam's brain to expect a fairly constant release of dopamine during his waking hours. It now occurs not only when Sam smokes, but even to some degree when Sam just thinks about smoking. Things that cause Sam to think about smoking, we call a "trigger". These triggers can include anything from being in a certain environment where Sam usually smokes, to being with friends who smoke, to experiencing stress, to getting just a little taste or whiff of cigarette smoke.

Sam may not understand triggers, but Sam's brain is nonetheless triggered, and dopamine is released just by thinking about smoking. So, Sam, despite his determination, has a deep fear his cravings will get so bad that he will panic and not be able to function unless his cigarettes are within his reach. Cigarettes have truly become Sam's best friend, in a very literal sense. Planning to avert disaster, Sam puts a single cigarette in his pocket as a safety net, so after he has thrown away his pack he will have a "back-up" if things get too terrible. To Sam this seems like a good idea, so he won't panic, as that seems to him to be a risk to cause him to relapse.

The next time Sam goes somewhere, he climbs into his car and notices the smell of the cigarettes in the car. Sam thinks of smoking then, whereupon he gets a small dopamine release (a trigger). Sam always loved to smoke while driving, so the act of driving causes him to think of a cigarette, and this results in another small dopamine release (a trigger). Sam is now driving along, and the rewards of smoking have already begun, but in smaller amounts. He is experiencing a "craving."

As the craving builds, Sam thinks of that cigarette in his pocket. He thinks of how wonderful it would be to light up that cigarette, which thought leads to a larger dopamine release, which is strongly reinforcing. So, without ever using the cigarette Sam has already experienced a large amount of reinforcing and rewarding dopamine release. He has experienced the cravings, the triggers, and an almost overwhelming need to get the rest of that dopamine release, while consciously telling himself he is going to stop smoking. It is too much for him, and so Sam reaches into his pocket, the action of doing so again triggering dopamine based on a behavioral trigger. After all, in the past when he has reached into his pocket he has soon had a dopamine reward for doing so.

Sam holds the cigarette in his fingers, feeling the familiar stiffness of the paper roll. He stares at his "safety net", telling himself he can stop, he can do this, while every moment of anticipation and contemplation leads to more dopamine release. He is glad that he has the cigarette in case it gets too bad, and he just can't make it without it. Finally, overwhelmed by his brain's chemical reward system, he lights up the cigarette, not able to withstand the thought of feeling the whole reward when the thing that would release all that dopamine is resting in his fingertips. The interesting thing is the amount of dopamine released after smoking the cigarette may not be significantly larger than what he was already experiencing, but it gave him that extra surge, and is certainly very reinforcing. The nicotine also calms his agitation, reinforcing it further.

This applies to many other behaviors as well—perhaps to any addictive behavior such as pornography, sexual indiscretion, drinking, or gambling. One day I sat down with a man who had been doing well after several years of being "clean" from a pornography addiction. He reported he is feeling really good. He feels the Spirit. When I asked about his pornography struggles he explained he still worried about the desire, but he found ways to combat that desire by listening to inspirational LDS speakers and doing other things that would bring the Spirit into his life. He had restrictions put into his life to remove access to pornography, and said he was so grateful for his lack of access. He then explained to me that the whole process of indulging in pornography didn't make sense to him.

One time he was caught looking at pornography. The very act had made him feel sick, and he hated it, even before he was caught. At the same time, there was such a powerful draw that he felt almost powerless to resist, despite his aversion to doing it. He still worried about his capacity to withstand the temptation, but had his focus on the peace and the joy received through a selection of different activities, particularly spiritually uplifting activities.

The role of dopamine and other neurotransmitters explains a great many of the destructive behaviors in which we find ourselves indulging. The role of these neurotransmitters applies directly to some of the more important laws the Lord has given us, specifically to the Word of Wisdom, the Law of Chastity, and the Ten Commandments. These laws of behavior, when uncontrolled, have had hugely devastating impacts in every era of our world's history. Many wars have been waged over wealth, power, the control of addictive substances, and even over the desire for the love of a woman.

The neurons and neurotransmitters in our body are very complex. The entire system is designed to maintain the functionality of this incredibly complex body we have. Neurotransmitters are key in the brain, but are also necessary in the rest of the body to send nerve signals to every part of our body. They are also very sensitive to change.

In order for our bodies to work correctly they must stay in balance. Balance comes at many levels. For example, the body needs to balance the acid in our body. First, there must be enough water in our body to act as a buffer, then the acid must be carefully controlled and excreted through our kidneys and lungs as uric acid or carbon dioxide. Such balance is also critical for the neurotransmitters. If neurotransmitters (such as serotonin) are out of balance, then we suffer from the imbalance (such as low serotonin levels leading to depression and anxiety).

One of the problems with drug abuse, physical trauma, stress, illness, sexual abuse, chronic disease, and other situations that impact our reward system is they throw off our balance. Drug use is an easy illustration. Most drugs of abuse cause a sudden extreme elevation or a prolonged elevation of dopamine within our brains. The reward to the mind seems amazing. However, once the dopamine has been depleted, withdrawal begins. Withdrawal is partially the result of not having enough dopamine in the synapse between the neurons. We then feel terrible and seek to feel good again.

The logical response is to use or do something the brain knows will stimulate more dopamine release. Normal activities no longer suffice because the dopamine release is not strong enough. When the dopamine supply in the brain is already depleted, it needs a stronger trigger to release more, and only the behavior or the drug being abused can make it happen. So, a pattern of repeat dosing begins, to regain that feeling of well-being: the drug is used; dopamine is released, but not as much as before, as the store of dopamine within the neuron has been depleted. This pattern is repeated until the actual mechanism of dopamine production and release is damaged. In some cases, such as with methamphetamine use, the dopamine producing cells can be damaged beyond function, or they can actually die, leaving the brain without the ability to produce sufficient dopamine.

If we think about the aircraft carrier, this is like destroying the radio. Let us say the plan did not go well, and the submarine evaded detection by the destroyer. The submarine fires a torpedo and hits the aircraft carrier. It was not a mortal wound, but chaos breaks out. Everyone is on alert, guns are firing, airplanes are launching, and the carrier has turned into mayhem, with every system in full alert and total overdrive. Every light is flashing, fires are raging, explosions are rocking the ship.

Because of the chaos, the crew cannot hear the radio. They turn up the volume on the radio so they can hear the destroyer and notify them of the distress. Suddenly another torpedo hits, and even more noise erupts. Once again, they turn up the volume of the radio, but this time they blow out the speakers. Now they have no means by which to communicate with anyone. They are helpless in the sea.

Though simplistic and not completely accurate relative to the methods of communication employed by a modern navy, this illustration may be helpful in understanding how critical neurotransmitters are for communication of signals in our brain. When we destroy those cells, or even damage them, our body and mind simply begin to fail in their function, like a listing aircraft carrier at sea.

To further comprehend the importance of the neurotransmitters, consider this about dopamine. Let us establish that a person who feels "normal" without any sort of artificial dopamine stimulation will be at 100% of a basal release of dopamine. (The "relative dopamine values" in the following charts have been adapted from data gathered from research on the effects of drugs on dopamine [2].) The times shown on the x-axis are estimates. The y-axis showing the intensity of the dopamine surge is the important value for this discussion. Dopamine is constantly being released in order to maintain our feeling of well-being along with many other very important functions, such as motor control (controlling our muscles).

Eating something delicious increases dopamine release to approximately 150% of normal for a brief period of time. That makes us feel good, reinforces our desire to eat again, and explains why we like to eat. Sex has a similar effect, but even more. With sex, we have a surge of about 200% of our normal dopamine levels (in other words, the dopamine in our brain doubles) but still only lasts for a short period of time (Fig. 1).

Drugs provide a release of dopamine similar to sex, yet often more prolonged. Morphine causes a dopamine high which continues for three or more hours (Fig. 2). This sustained release

Fig. 1

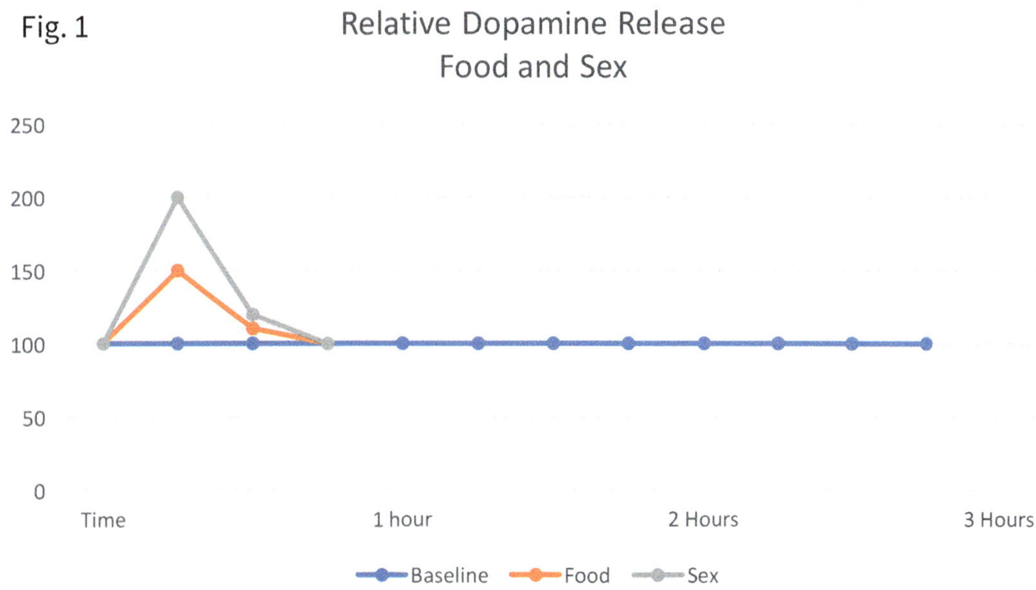

of dopamine from morphine, with the ongoing euphoria, explains some of the addictive potential of the drug. Of course, some people do not like the way it makes them feel, primarily because of the way their body metabolizes morphine. Many users become nauseated when morphine breaks down into codeine in their system. Others are less lucky, and thoroughly enjoy the prolonged intense dopamine release. These are the people most likely to become addicted.

Other drugs are similar, but often trigger a dopamine release even more intense than morphine. Nicotine, for example, causes high, short acting peaks of dopamine (Fig 3). This results in rapid and repeated reinforcement as smokers have to smoke frequently to maintain the dopamine effect (Fig. 4). This, along with many other factors (including being legal, socially accepted, easily accessible, relatively inexpensive, etc.) helps make nicotine one of the most addictive drugs, and one of the most dangerous and expensive of societies' drug problems.

Alcohol affects many neurotransmitters and reward systems. It does affect dopamine in addition to many other pathways, and its effects are measurable. The following graphs (Figs. 5 and 6) shows the dopamine effects derived from ethanol (alcohol) and cocaine.

Note that dopamine release from ethanol (alcohol) does not go as high as some of the other drugs. However, it is involved with so many other reward pathways that it is highly reinforcing. In this particular graph, one can see the intense dopamine levels triggered by cocaine, the stimulant derived from Coca leaves that made Coca-Cola a worldwide phenomenon before the cocaine was removed from the drink in 1903. Of course, cocaine has also been manipulated into "crack cocaine" that can be smoked, providing an incredibly rapid delivery to the brain, which would be much faster than reflected in the Figure 6. It is also more addicting and perhaps more intense in the dopamine release in the "crack" form.

Fig. 2

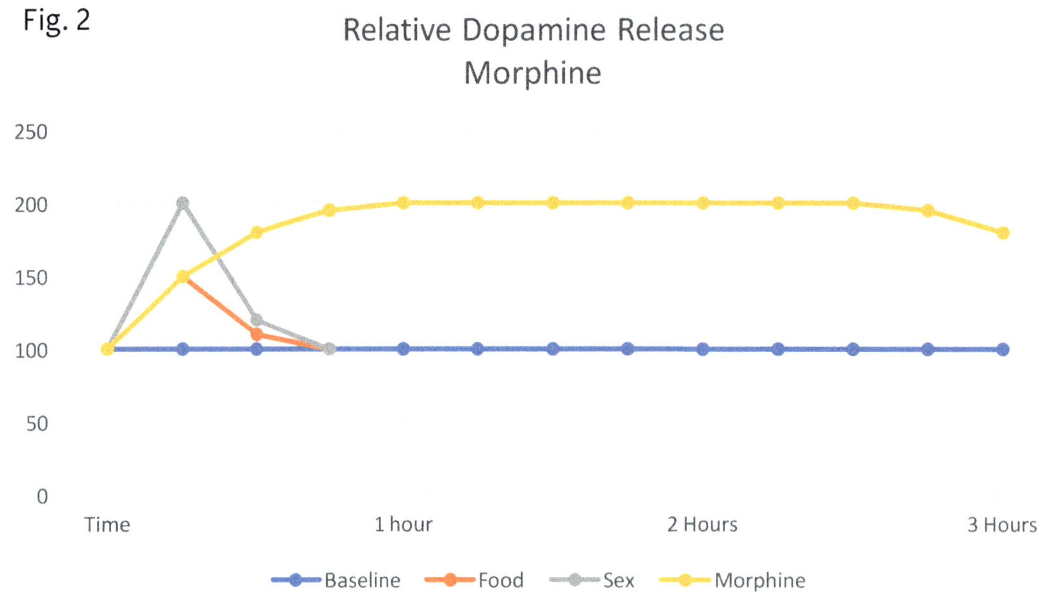
Relative Dopamine Release
Morphine
250
200
150
100
50
0
Time
1 hour
2 Hours
3 Hours
Baseline
Food
Sex
Morphine

Fig. 3

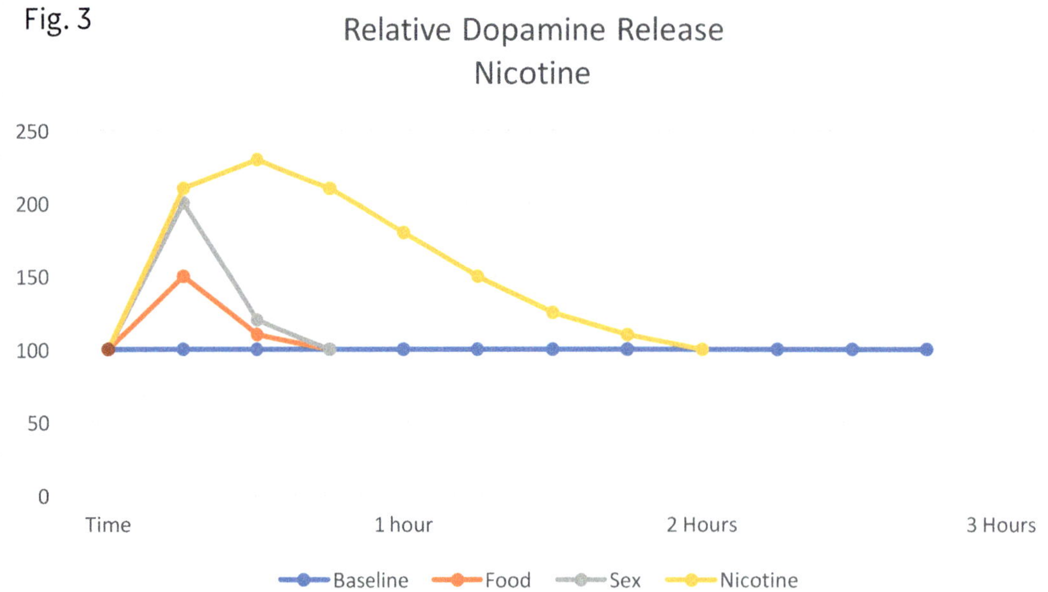
Relative Dopamine Release
Nicotine
250
200
150
100
50
0
Time
1 hour
2 Hours
3 Hours
Baseline
Food
Sex
Nicotine

Fig. 4

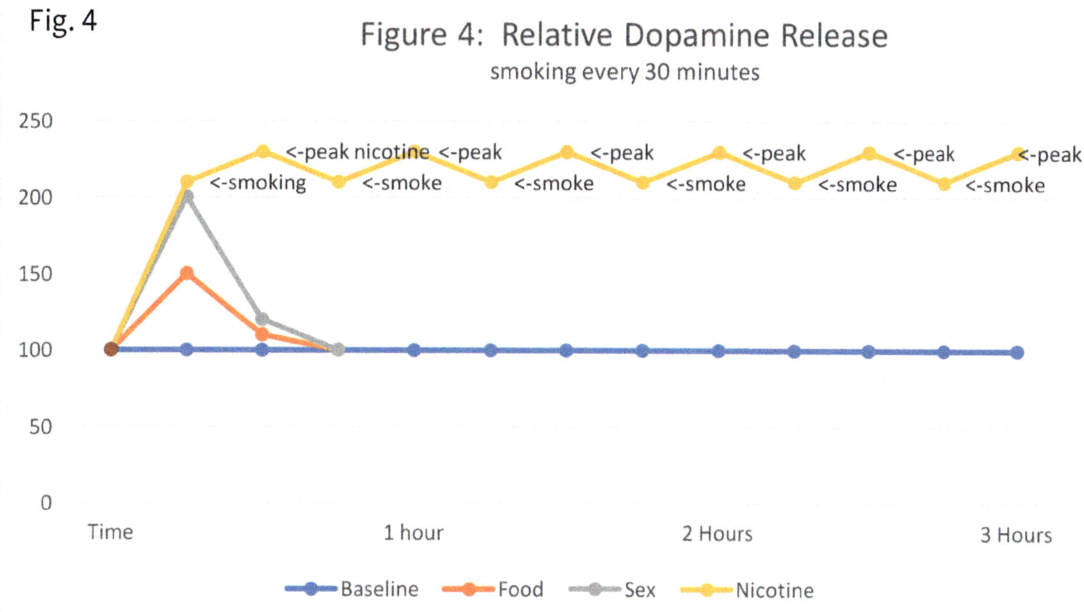
Figure 4: Relative Dopamine Release
smoking every 30 minutes
250
200
150
100
50
0
<-peak nicotine
<-peak
<-peak
<-peak
<-peak
<-peak
<-smoking
<-smoke
<-smoke
<-smoke
<-smoke
<-smoke
Time
1 hour
2 Hours
3 Hours
Baseline
Food
Sex
Nicotine

Fig. 5

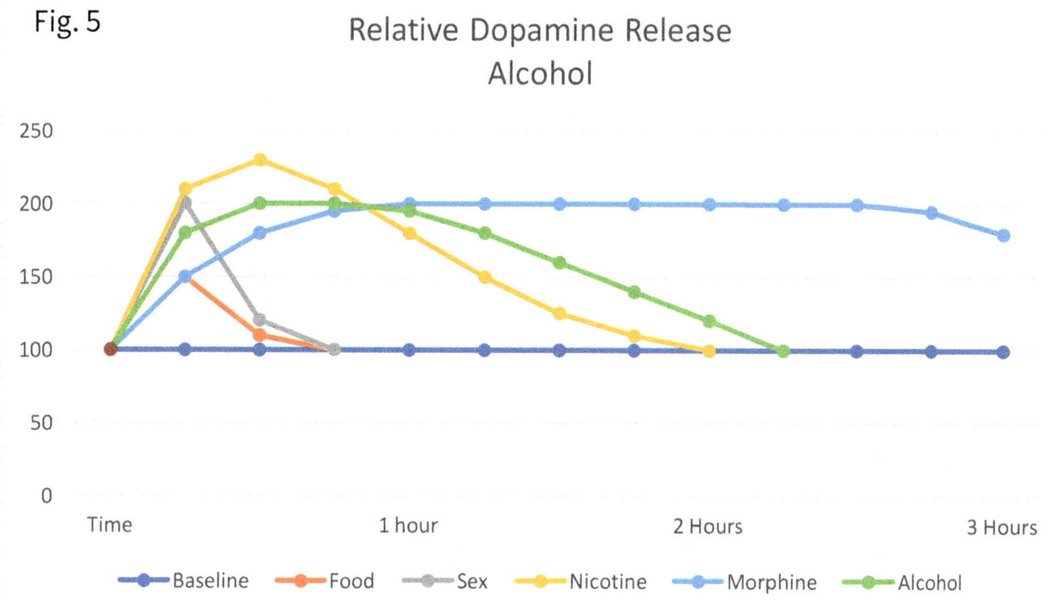
Relative Dopamine Release
Alcohol
250
200
150
100
50
0
Time
1 hour
2 Hours
3 Hours
Baseline
Food
Sex
Nicotine
Morphine
Alcohol

Fig. 6

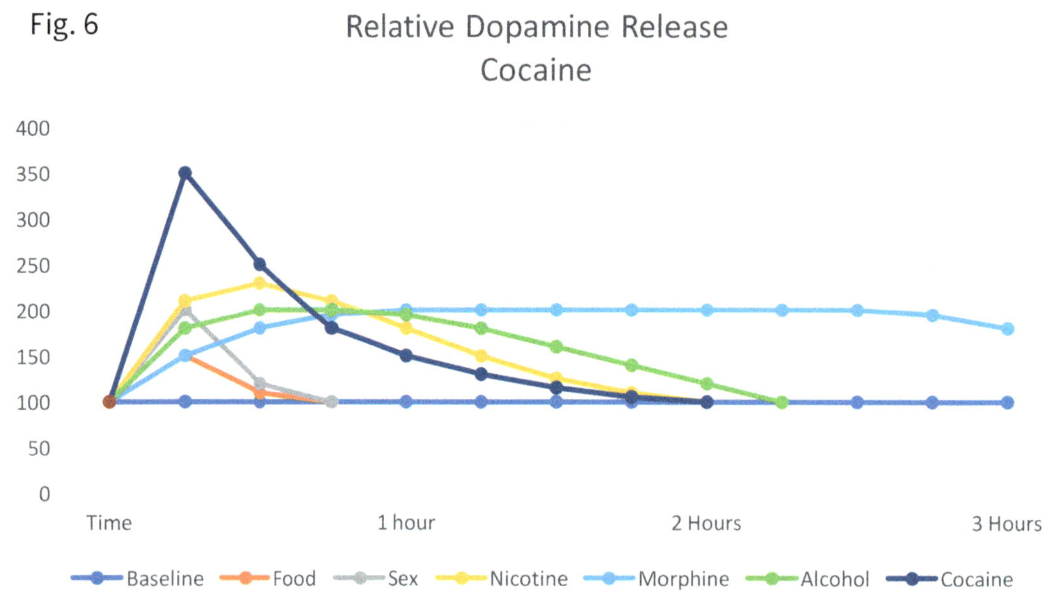

Then we have methamphetamine. Often referred to as Meth, this drug was developed in 1919 and used extensively during World War II to enhance soldiers' energy, alertness, and effectiveness in combat. It was abandoned after the war due to bad side effects, but then re-discovered in the 1960's with the extensive drug experimentation of that era. It can be refined into a very pure substance, and has become a devastating drug of abuse. Figure 7 shows why.

The dopamine release from methamphetamine dwarfs the dopamine from every other drug and behavior. The dopamine released from using meth hits 1000% of the basal dopamine levels. I once heard a lecturing addiction specialist refer to this as "a nuclear bomb in the brain." I think that is an appropriate description. This not only overwhelms the brain with an artificial chemical high, but it severely depletes dopamine stores. Meth is one of those drugs which people rapidly seek again simply to avoid the severe dopamine deficiency that follows.

The graphic depiction of dopamine release shown in the graphs in this chapter help us understand several concepts about dopamine as a neurotransmitter. First, at normal levels derived from pleasurable activities such as eating, it works as a good reward system, to help us want to repeat that pleasurable activity. At those levels, it also does not deplete dopamine, so that we do not have a withdrawal phase, and we can continue to have normal dopamine responses to that same activity in the future.

Second, drugs that stimulate artificial elevations or prolongations of dopamine do result in dopamine depletion. This is partly why drug users begin to develop withdrawals and cravings to use again. In extreme cases, such as methamphetamines, the nerve cells which produce dopamine are actually damaged or destroyed, resulting in permanent damage to the brain's reward system.

Fig. 7

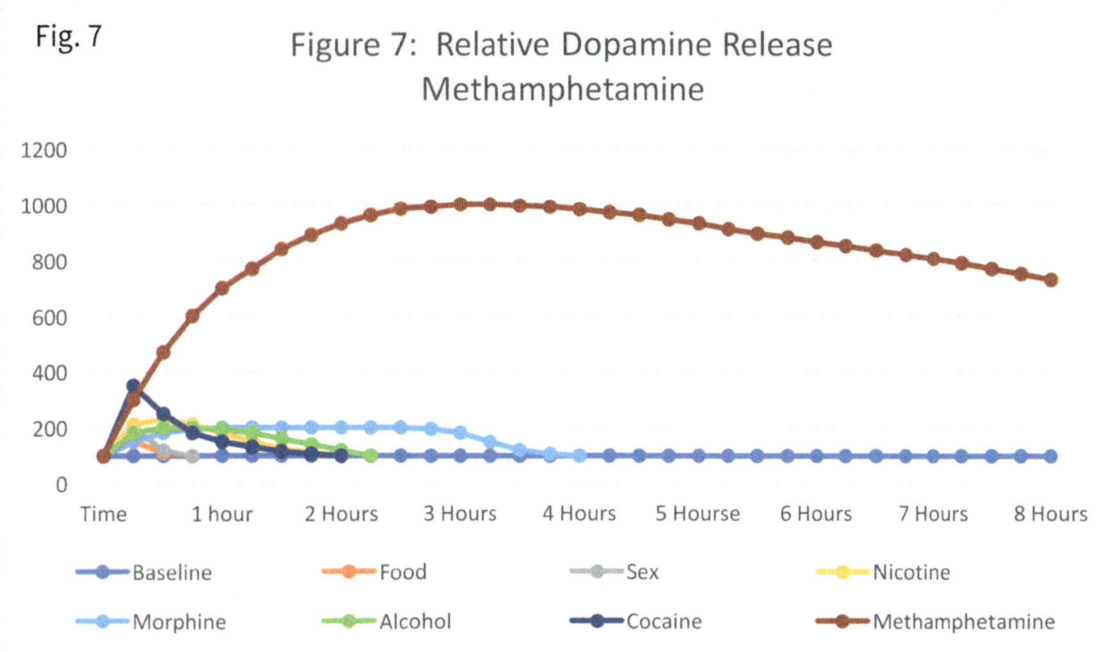

For example, some people who abuse methamphetamine develop health conditions very similar to Parkinson's Disease, which is the result of neurons not having enough dopamine.

Third, the body wants to get back to normal. Referring back to the example of the aircraft carrier, as soon as the speakers on the aircraft carrier blow out, the admiral sends for repair men to get them fixed. The brain does the same. In the case of neurotransmitters, there are several mechanisms. The neurons begin to more rapidly reabsorb the neurotransmitter from the synapse. The neurons also begin to remove or disable the receptors that are triggered by the neurotransmitters. These processes are what lead to tolerance to drugs, so the drugs have less effect even though the same amount is used. This process of downgrading receptors and reducing the quantity of neurotransmitters also leads to dependence, meaning that if the drug is stopped, the body suddenly does not have enough neurotransmitters to function normally, and withdrawals occur.

Despite the simplicity of the illustrations in this chapter, the neurotransmitter concept is key to understanding addiction. However, different drugs affect different neurotransmitters, and different neurotransmitters have different effects in the brain. Thus, we see the amazing variance in drug effects, from the mild stimulation of caffeine to the overwhelming and destructive euphoria of methamphetamine.

Neurotransmitters appear to be the key to understanding the addiction process, as well as the key for our ability in the future to treat addictions more successfully. Medical treatments will revolve around stabilizing neurotransmitter levels. Behavioral treatments will also likely be much enhanced once we understand better the interaction of all the chemicals within the brain, allowing us to understand how and why our brains and bodies respond the way they do.

CHAPTER 6

Is Addiction A Disease?

"Medical research describes addiction as "a disease of the brain." This is true, but I believe that once Satan has someone in his grasp, it also becomes a disease of the spirit."

Elder M. Russell Ballard [1]

As we further discuss issues relating to neurotransmitters and addiction, we must review the model of addiction as a disease. This is very often a point of contention and disagreement. For centuries, societies embraced the idea that addicts were simply people of weak character or moral depravity. Fortunately, as we learn more about addiction, we are building a different model. The American Society of Addiction Medicine (ASAM) takes the position that addiction follows the same model as other chronic disease processes. Many people disagree and feel addiction is simply a behavioral problem.

Much of what is fueling the current debate over addiction being a disease or not stems from our current health care model. Right now our health care delivery is controlled by "third party payers," otherwise known as insurance companies, medicare, and medicaid. If addiction is classified as a disease then these payers are under greater obligation to pay for treatment for addiction. This could create all sorts of debates regarding who is paying, if tax dollars are being used, and much more. It is not my intent to discuss the political issues surrounding payment and treatment. Even so, I think it is very useful to understand the debate about addiction as a disease. Despite the feelings one may have about the politics of health care, there is a certainty: Addiction is on the rise. It is now the leading cause of death in Americans under the age of 50 years old. It is the biggest portion of accidental deaths, and accidental deaths are the 4th leading cause of death in the United States. Addiction is closely associated with mental health. However we approach the treatment of addiction, we have to realize that we need to begin addressing it soon, as addiction and mental health are beginning to consume our resources and severely tax our society. This will likely only get worse.

We have discussed many ways and examples in which addictive behaviors follow the same chemical pathways and utilize the same neurotransmitters as do chemical addictions. Persisting reinforcement of these behaviors makes it ever more difficult to maintain our agency. Over time the abuse of these chemical pathways changes our perspective and leads to the loss of personal impulse control, the loss of our freedoms, and eventually we give away our agency because we begin to lose our ability to choose otherwise without severe physical and emotional suffering.

Chemical addiction can become even more of a physical disease, as it goes beyond the modification of chemical pathways by repeated behaviors. The introduction of foreign chemical compounds into our body actually changes the structure and function of our body. The body is designed to maintain a balance, known as "homeostasis." If something is introduced which upsets that balance, then the body compensates, changing its own structure or function to compensate for the changes to avoid illness or death.

Interestingly, with modern scanning technology we can study the structure and function of the brain. Drug-induced changes within the brain are clearly identifiable. Some of these changes become permanent. Yet, in people who are more at risk for addiction, similar structural changes may already exist that pre-date the use of toxic chemicals and drugs. Some changes are not as visible relative to structural changes in the brain. However, functional imaging is showing similar findings.

For example, opiates change the function, structure, and composition of our own internal naturally-produced opiate system. Over time, the artificial administration of opiates to the body causes the body to quit making its own opiates for pain control. It also causes the body to remove opiate receptors from the post-synaptic neurons so that opiates within the synapses will have less effect. This explains the primary process by which we develop tolerance, dependence, withdrawal, and addiction to opiates.

Alcohol changes the function and structure of almost every organ and chemical system in our body. Not only does it trigger or inhibit most reward systems that we now understand, it also physically damages almost every tissue in the body to which it is exposed.

Methamphetamine, bath salts, spice, and other "designer" drugs simply destroy tissues (particularly in the brain, and most particularly in developing brains), thus irreversibly altering our physical, mental, and emotional balance.

These scenarios meet the definition of chronic disease in that the structure and function of our bodies has been altered and no longer function normally.

Chronic disease models are more successful in treating illnesses such as diabetes, heart disease, and kidney disease. This is true for many reasons. With a chronic disease model, we are able to have better long-term follow up. We are also able to more effectively address the issues relative to genetic predisposition or environmental impact. It is difficult to truly sort out whether many of these diseases are primarily genetic or environmental. This may not sound too important, but the study of addiction has shown that genetic predispositions do have a huge impact on both the development and the treatment of a disease process.

We know many illnesses are primarily genetic and we are born with them, and will likely experience some degree of their effect within our lifetime. Examples could include the following: Type 1 diabetes (juvenile onset), familial hyperlipidemia (high cholesterols and/or triglycerides), Alport's Syndrome (a genetic familial kidney disease leading to kidney failure, blindness, and deafness followed by premature death), and Down's Syndrome (Trisomy 21). Some cancers develop simply from genetic defects and mutations. A myriad of other things we inherit (including susceptibility to chemical addictions such as alcoholism) very easily lead to long-term problems. Identification of specific genes which carry those traits may be very important in the prevention of such diseases.

Some genetically predisposed illnesses may be preventable with the appropriate life decisions, but can be a high risk for us even if we work hard to avoid them. Type II diabetes, strokes, and cardiovascular disease are good examples of a combination of multiple risk factors, any one of which could lead to the disease, including high cholesterol, high blood pressure, type A personalities, etc. Renal failure is another example which could be the end product of either genetic conditions, environmental factors, or combinations of both.

Some diseases are almost entirely induced by environmental or behavioral factors. Rheumatic heart disease is caused by untreated strep infections. Secondary renal failure (such as that caused by uncontrolled diabetes, dehydration, drug use, extensive use of anti-inflammatories, etc.) is an example of chronic disease brought on by other diseases. Strokes and cardiovascular disease can be caused by overeating or eating the wrong foods, inactive lifestyles, smoking, alcohol abuse, etc., and are all examples of diseases that can be brought upon ourselves even without strong genetic predispositions. Elephantiasis is a very destructive parasitic disease of the lymphatic system and is completely externally imposed. Venereal diseases are primarily self-imposed and take a willful act to acquire them (with the exceptions of abuse, rape, and other violent crimes) but have no genetic predisposition (unless we consider mental illness as a genetic factor).

The above examples are quite simplistic, but show some of the futility of trying to claim something is a disease only if it is not self-inflicted, or is not a disease simply because it was self-inflicted. To bring this into further focus, we are reminded many of the diseases on which we spend most of our money are diseases that could be modified and even controlled with lifestyle, meaning self-control and good choices. For example:

1. Heart disease.
2. Lung disease (smoking)
3. Accidents (including overdose)
4. Stroke
5. Diabetes
6. Influenza and pneumonia
7. Obesity related illness

The list could go on. In fact, simply take a look at the list on the following page of leading causes of death in the United States from 2013 and note how many of them can be modified by behavioral management.

One of the most dramatic health crises in America right now is the rise of obesity and the myriad of health problems which it causes. Again, many will argue that there is a genetic predisposition to obesity. However, if that were the biggest factor, then obesity would have been just as

The 15 leading causes of death in 2013 were: [2]

1. Diseases of heart (heart disease)
2. Malignant neoplasms (cancer)
3. Chronic lower respiratory diseases
4. Accidents (unintentional injuries)
5. Cerebrovascular diseases (stroke)
6. Alzheimer's disease
7. Diabetes mellitus (diabetes)
8. Influenza and pneumonia
9. Nephritis, nephrotic syndrome and nephrosis (kidney disease)
10. Intentional self-harm (suicide)
11. Septicemia
12. Chronic liver disease and cirrhosis
13. Essential hypertension and hypertensive renal dis ease (hypertension)
14. Parkinson's disease
15. Pneumonitis due to solids and liquids

large a problem for our ancestors. We now simply have to accept that our epidemic of obesity is primarily related to several things:

1. Poor choices in diet and lifestyle (activity levels).
2. Lack of self-control (ability to practice moderation).
3. Being addicted to the body's chemical reward system for eating (in the same sense that we have discussed with other behavioral and chemical addictions).
4. Genetic predisposition to obesity due to dysfunction of the inhibitory and reward systems related to eating.

These factors are manifest in a general nation-wide lack of physical activity, overeating, and poor dietary choices, based on choosing that which is delicious, pleasant and most enjoyable (physical appetites, the "Natural Man") rather than that which is most healthy. With obesity as an example of similar factors that lead to heart disease, strokes, some cancers, diabetic complications, and many other diseases, it is hard to say we must eliminate self-inflicted ailments from our list of diseases simply because we bring them upon ourselves. However, we should also encourage a system which requires more accountability when we commit time and resources to any of these individuals who choose not to make good decisions regarding their own health.

A reflection upon the history of addiction treatment is quite interesting from the perspective of how we perceive addiction in our society. The Latin derivation of the word addiction is addicere, and means "enslaved by" or "bound to". At first this was used to refer to behavioral disorders, not drug disorders. Addiction then began to be applied to alcohol abuse and over time it was applied to other drugs of abuse. Only within the past couple of decades has it been accepted once again as a description of behavioral disorders (such as eating disorders, gambling disorders, etc). [3]

A review of some of the things predisposing a person to addiction also reflects the concept that addiction is more deeply-seated than simply being the result of one or two bad decisions. Psychiatric disorders often contribute to or lead to drug abuse and drug addiction. Not only is this true in general, but specific types of psychiatric illness are much more closely linked with certain types of addictions. Functional scanning of the brain shows many people with psychiatric illness who have never used drugs have similar scans to those who have abused drugs. In other words, some people's brains simply do not function normally to begin with, and if they ever use a drug that compensates for that deficiency then they finally feel normal and want to continue with the drug. This is a factor that is certainly beyond the simple explanation of bad moral judgment, or even choice. They did not choose to have a brain that functions sub-optimally. However, it also cannot be the excuse to justify issues over which the individual still does have agency. Additionally, certain types of brain injuries may lead to a higher risk of addiction, probably through loss of a specific function within the brain. In the case of addiction, this could be a direct effect upon the neurotransmitters in the reward system.

Other indicators can help us understand addiction as a chronic disease. Family histories are extremely useful for anticipating potential addiction problems. This would mean there is more to addiction than just poor morals. We know addiction is not solely due to family culture or common environments (though those factors have a large influence), because studies on twins separated at birth show similar addictive tendencies.

At one conference, I listened to an expert give a lecture on alcohol addiction. She noted a family history was very predictive of alcoholism in families—except in Mormons, as they did not show consistent alcoholism problems because so many of them do not drink. This, or course, highlights the potential power environmental influences and choices can have in the process of addiction. We do know genetic predisposition does exist in Mormons just like anyone else, as those who do drink seem to have the same risk of addiction as non-Mormons. It is just not a cultural norm to take the risk. On the other hand, we do not know how genetic predisposition affects people before they ever try a drink. Could it be that those Mormons who choose to drink (or have any other addiction) have genetic influences that put them at higher risk before ever being exposed, and perhaps even a higher risk of being exposed? This could include individual ways in which we deal with stress, or family environments, or psychiatric illness, etc.

Some have pointed to the idea that addiction is not a disease based on the tendency for relapse, which seems to be a behavioral issue. They feel if it were truly a disease, then treatment would be curative. If a qualification of being a disease process were to be curative then most cancers would not be considered a disease, as few cancers are truly curable at this time. Nor would heart disease, arthritis, or Parkinson's Disease. Additionally, if the characteristic of relapse removes an illness from being a disease process, then anyone who goes back to the office with elevated blood sugars and uncontrolled diabetes because they are not complying with their diet, or worsening blood pressure because they quit exercising, could not be considered to have a chronic disease. Relapse, progression, and having to retake control of the disease process are all routine characteristics of any chronic disease. These are also characteristics of mortality, and drawing nearer to that final exit event called death.

In recent years, the same debate has surrounded depression and other psychiatric illnesses. Depression is being more and more accepted as a chronic disease. However, this has not been the case for very long. In the past many felt people with depression just needed to "pull themselves up by the bootstraps," or to just "get it together and quit doing things that cause depression." Other psychiatric illnesses have likewise been viewed as just bad behavior and poor choices. Again, brain scans clearly show structural and functional differences in the brains of people with psychiatric illness, just as with addictions. I do believe depression and other psychologic illness can be the outcome of choosing to live contrary to the teachings of Jesus Christ, or the outcome of addictive behaviors. We simply cannot turn our back on the Light of Christ, and the knowledge we have from the pre-existence, to pursue our own carnal desires and self-gratification without suffering depression. However, I believe many who live righteous and wonderful lives do suffer depression due to dysfunctions of their brain and the imbalance of chemicals and neurotransmitters.

In a landmark talk in October of 2013, Elder Jeffrey R. Holland said the following: "I wish to speak to those who suffer from some form of mental illness or emotional disorder, whether those afflictions be slight or severe, of brief duration or persistent over a lifetime. We sense the complexity of such matters when we hear professionals speak of neurosis and psychoses, of genetic predispositions and chromosome defects, of bipolarity, paranoia, and schizophrenia. However, bewildering this all may be, these afflictions are some of the realities of mortal life, and there should be no more shame in acknowledging them than in acknowledging a battle with high blood pressure or the sudden appearance of a malignant tumor." [4]

With the same sense of compassion which Elder Holland expressed in that talk, can we not also look at the addict with such compassion? From a mortal perspective, it may sometimes be difficult to explain or to understand such complex issues. However, from a Christ-like perspective, perhaps we can look at addiction as we do mental illness, realizing every person is unique, not only in their challenges and trials, but in their capacity to handle those challenges and trials. Perhaps we can accept what is not a hardship for one person may be a terrible burden for another person, rather than simply a "moral flaw." Perhaps we can also see that the physical differences of our mortal bodies, one from another, help explain our different susceptibilities to these challenges.

Ultimately, we are mortal, and subject to all the potential mutations and deteriorations of genetics over the past 6,000 years, in addition to all the environmental pressures of our highly toxic environment. Everyone suffers with terminal mortal failings. Some people's bodies suffer from disease. Some people's minds suffer from disease. Some have a combination. There are so many different ways these are manifest that the most rigorous students of the human body still struggle with the complexity of its workings, trying to identify, label and learn to heal those things which we still don't understand well.

Having said that, we have to be very careful no one interprets this as an excuse to give up and say their genetic and environmental influences have made it impossible to overcome addiction. We can overcome addiction because, unlike some other diseases, it is not innately fatal. Eventually heart disease and diabetes are fatal because they are the progression of aging and dying bodies. The only part of addiction that is fatal is the continued use of the substance, or the persistence of the behavior. Our focus needs to be on finding models of treatment that are more effective, and on preventing or avoiding addiction altogether.

Applying the model of chronic disease does have a major benefit for us beyond simply the political and payment implications. We have already seen treatment models which have been very effective in treating addiction. These models have been built around recovery programs for nurses, physicians, lawyers, and airline pilots. Theses models are more consistent with treatment that reflects a chronic disease model of care. They often consisted of longer treatment programs, but the real key may be that they have much more structured follow up. Such models have shown high rates of successful sobriety after many years. Certainly one could argue the greater success rate is attributable to the fact that these individuals careers are at stake, and to maintain their licenses they are required to stay sober. This is an interesting argument, since the very nature of addiction shows that people lose careers and other important components of their lives due to their addictions. Perhaps there are other factors. However, gaining leverage to maintain long-term follow up seems to be a critical component of maintaining recovery.

We are also seeing more programs which gather a team of specialists, representing behavioral medicine, psychiatric medicine, addiction medicine, and social work, with other available resources to consult on and determine the most appropriate treatment for individual clients. The hope is that such treatment programs tailored to each individual client will not only aid in the recovery of that individual, but help assure more consistent follow up for those individuals.

In summary, the model of addiction as a chronic disease is important to understand as it may open the way for more successful treatment programs. Just as we know that if we do not follow-up regularly with patients who have diseases such as diabetes and hypertension, they tend to lose control of their disease over time, success in addiction treatment may be largely dependent on our ability to maintain consistent follow-up. Changing the way we think about addiction will help change the model of treatment to be more consistent with the way we treat other chronic diseases.

CHAPTER 7

Risk Factors for Addiction

"Society has made a great effort to modernize the world in education, communication, travel, health, commerce, housing, and in many other ways, so as to increase the standard of living; but what has this socialization and modernization done to the family—the basic institution of society? Never before has there been greater instability... Drug addiction, disobedience to law, increase in venereal disease, and corruption in all forms seem to be accepted... Surely we would agree that the family institution has been seriously, if not irreparably, damaged in our society."

Howard W. Hunter [1]

Science continually studies and tries to identify the risk factors for addiction, in the hopes of being able to prevent addiction. Much has been discovered about the genetics and physiology behind addiction. There are many other factors behind addiction, and defining them all seems to be an endless task.

As quoted above, Howard W. Hunter (and many other leaders) have been warning us for decades of a terrible risk: the destruction of the family as the primary arena for teaching and protecting our children from spiritual destruction. Whereas this chapter will focus on many of the identifiable risks for addiction, we should also realize the loss of the core family unit is really a key component (perhaps the key component) in trying to quantify all of these risks. Such destabilization of the family leads to an inevitable loss of our moral foundations, and though we spend decades and billions of dollars trying to identify and avert the risk factors for society's ills, these efforts will be in vain until we rebuild our families and regain a solid moral foundation. Without this, society will continue to crumble.

In 1971 Elder N. Eldon Tanner said the following: "Again we might ask: Where am I when it comes to teaching my family, by example as well as by precept, to walk uprightly before the Lord, to be honest and honorable in all their dealings…? Am I aware of the increasing availability of illegal drugs, and warning my children of the dangers involved? What am I doing in my community to clear up problems pertaining to drug addiction, alcoholism, sexual promiscuity and disease, which are more prevalent than most parents realize?" [2]

Without strong families, the list of "risk factors" found for addiction will continue to grow, and we will continue to struggle unsuccessfully to find a solution to those risk factors. The greatest safety is in teaching our children, in a family setting, to believe in Christ and live a Christ-centered life.

Spiritually, we could certainly argue there are many factors, such as intemperance, pride, lack of obedience, and lack of self-discipline. We will forever be confronted with the ongoing debate of "nature versus nurture" as we discuss risks for behavioral and medical problems. That is simply a discussion trying to sort out how much of who we are is because of our genetics, and how much of it is because of our environment.

The difficulty of this discussion, and the reason it will never be fully answered, is because the third component which is never given recognition in that scientific discussion is the spiritual component—who we were before we ever obtained a physical body. We know much of who we are now already existed in the pre-mortal realm (who we were before birth). We are still that spiritual being whom God created, who learned and grew and became a spirit who chose to follow Christ during the pre-mortal council in heaven. Even at that time we had faith. We decided we would be obedient to God's plan. All of us who are on earth now, actually chose the difficulty and test of mortality over the lie of an easy life and supposedly guaranteed salvation at the hands of Lucifer. He proposed we use our agency to give up our agency, with the promise of forcing us to be obedient, and saving every one of us (despite the impossibility of being able to force anyone to perfection). It was impossible to do so, for it is only through acting on our own agency, choosing the better path, and living in accordance with a Celestial law of our own free will and choice, that we can become perfect like God.

Therefore, we chose in the pre-mortal realm to follow Christ. Those of us who accepted the difficulty of mortality came with the spiritual growth which would allow us to feel and recognize the Light of Christ, and to be able to follow the Holy Spirit to complete our missions here on this earth.

However, our trials come because our Spirits are placed in mortal bodies, and we become subject to all the appetites, passions, and desires of the flesh: the "Natural Man." In addition to this, we each have a completely different environment in which we are raised and live. The promise to us, however, is whatever our physical or environmental circumstances, the Spirit of the Lord can be with us if we allow Him. God has shown us how to do that, through obedience to the teachings of Christ, through faith and repentance, and renewing our covenants each week with the Sacrament. Then we can enjoy the guidance of the Holy Spirit.

So, how can it just be a matter of nature versus nurture? The real question in our discussion of risk factors for addiction is our desire and effort to open our spiritual self to the guidance and promptings of the Holy Ghost. He will lead us, teach us, guide us, and bring all things to our remembrance. He will also lead others who are following the Lord to teach us, guide us, and bear us up in our trials.

A member of my family grew up in an environment of drugs and in the absence of stable parental role models. Yet this individual followed the feelings of the Light of Christ, and as a teenager chose to be baptized. Despite trials and challenges beyond what many will ever see or understand, this individual has served a mission, married in the temple, and is raising a family in faith, with the Spirit and the priesthood in their home. That is the true safety, and is the biggest influence in our development, and in our risks for addiction (or sin of any sort). Our receptiveness and dependence on our Savior will be the deciding factor, more than any questions of nature or nurture.

However, simply being human is an almost overwhelming risk factor. We are subject to the flesh. And while our appetites, passions and desires can be good, and are essential to our survival, they are also the potential path to our destruction. No one is immune. We must either control them, avoid them, or pass through the extreme pain of regaining control of them once they have begun to control us.

The physical and environmental risks of addiction are multi-factorial, and often very confusing. Many stereotypes exist regarding who is a "druggie" or who is going to become an addict. Research has identified many risk factors for addiction that seem to depend on three different systems: the nature of the addictive substance, the environment, and the individual's genetics.

Every substance has its positive and negative effects. Every individual has their own sense of what "feels good." However, studies have been done with rats to see how many times a rat is willing to hit a button in order to get a dose of a specific drug. This "hit" scale is a good indicator of which substances stimulate the reward system more, and are thus more addictive. Again, every individual is different, and some substances are less rewarding for one individual than for another. As a general rule this scale seems to be fairly accurate at indicating the addictive potential of any particular substance.

Environmental factors also play a large role. Certain jobs expose individuals to drugs on a regular basis. Peer groups influence our youth to a huge degree. Some studies indicate that parental influence drops to 10% of the youth's environmental influence by age fourteen. The other 90% of the influence comes from forces outside the home, primarily peers. Some cultures teach abstinence while some teach tolerance, and yet others fully embrace the use of substances such as alcohol or hallucinogens from an early age. In such cases the risk of addiction is dramatically increased, as evidence clearly shows a much higher risk of addiction when any potentially addictive substance is used at an earlier age. Social instabilities such as poverty or peer rejection also lead to seeking an escape through substance use. Sexual abuse is also a predictable and large factor in women's risk for addiction, particularly sexual abuse before adolescence.

Genetics, of course, cannot be ignored. As has been shown over and over, many addiction disorders run in families, such as alcoholism. Different races also have different capacities to tolerate drugs. For example, Caucasians metabolize alcohol much more efficiently than most Asians.

Therefore, an Asian is more likely to become ill from the effects of alcohol earlier than a Caucasian. Based on the concepts of addictive potential, this puts the Caucasian at a higher risk for becoming addicted to alcohol than an Asian. This, in fact, helps dispel a myth that it is better if one can "hold their liquor". The real fact is individuals who can tolerate a large amount of alcohol are at much greater risk for developing alcoholism than those who cannot tolerate alcohol. Women also have less capacity to handle alcohol than men, due to less of an enzyme called alcohol dehydrogenase that helps break down alcohol. If they cannot tolerate the presence of the alcohol, then it is very difficult to develop a tolerance for it, and therefore they are less likely to become addicted to it.

Finally, individuals with psychiatric illness seem to be much more prone to drug abuse disorders. Current evidence suggests that often these individuals are attempting to self-medicate their illness by using the substances. This can include a host of problems, including attention deficit disorder, depression, bipolar disorder, personality disorders, schizophrenia, etc. Sometimes, however, after years of drug use it is difficult to ascertain whether the mental illness led to the addiction or the addiction led to the mental illness.

A good resource for more in-depth discussion of risk factors for addiction is ASAM's Textbook, *Principles of Addiction Medicine.*[3]

AGENT RELATED:

Availability

Individuals who have easy access to the addictive substance or behavior are more likely to become addicted, simply because they are more likely to experiment with something that is readily available and generally accepted. In many cases, the availability also reflects a cultural attitude about that substance or behavior. For example, parents who drink or smoke are sometimes prone to give their children "samples" at young ages, and are not as likely to be concerned about it when their children begin to use that substance themselves. This unfortunately leads to a higher chance that those children will have addiction problems as adults.

Parents who make meth or sell opiates are likely to share drugs or use drugs along with their children at some point. Children who see their parents gambling will often accept gambling as a normal part of adulthood, and an acceptable social norm. Availability may not be perceived by the adult, and abuse or addiction may end up being an unintended consequence, as we know that at least 66% of the abused prescription opiates come from a friend or family member just trying to "help out."

Other factors strongly affect availability. For example, for many decades opiates (like morphine) were considered unacceptable, with laws restricting them, patients fearing them, and physicians refusing to prescribe them. At the end of the 20th century opiates became more acceptable as they were found to be very beneficial in treating patients with cancer pain and providing end of life relief in patients dying from extremely painful illnesses. This use was extrapolated to other chronic pain syndromes. Suddenly there began to be media coverage on "under-treated pain." Legal actions were taken against doctors who were not "adequately" treating their patients. Pain management with opiates became the standard, accepted and expected treatment for chronic pain. In addition, hospitals were penalized for not controlling patients' pain. The unfortunate result has been a shocking and dramatic increase in prescription opiate abuse during the first decade of the 21st century. Now America is being overwhelmed with prescription opiate abuse and addiction.

Cost

Certainly, cost affects availability. This is clearly a factor in the more popular drugs we see being used. The resurgence of heroin is due to the cheaper production outstripping some of the more expensive prescription opiates. As prescription opiates become more difficult to obtain via cost shifting and regulatory restriction, heroin is once again a common street addiction.

Methamphetamine use surged when large Mexican labs took over mass production (and therefore cheap production). It rose again when stateside production in "meth houses" increased the local availability and decreased the cost.

Part of instituting taxes on tobacco and alcohol is not only to generate revenue to offset the societal cost of their use, but also to create a real disincentive to use them, and it works.

Rapidity With Which the Agent Reaches the Brain

The faster a substance reaches the brain, the more addictive it is. Taking pills orally is the slowest, and least popular, taking 15–30 minutes for most compounds to take effect. Taken in pill form, the drug usually absorbs in the stomach, transfers through the blood from the gut and passes through the liver, which "detoxifies" much of it. After it is thus slowly absorbed through the gut and then largely removed by the liver it has to find its way across the "blood-brain barrier", a very effective structure that keeps many of the things in our normal circulation from reaching our brain.

Other routes of drug use avoid passing through the liver, which avoids that first chance for the body to detoxify the substance before it can reach the brain. Snorting and injecting are much faster than the oral route, taking only minutes to reach the brain. Inhalation of vapors is also very rapid, very dangerous, and very addicting. The compounds being inhaled reach the brain by way of absorption through lung tissues as rapidly as 7 seconds. This is not only quick, but the dose is generally large, and very potent, giving an intense, though brief, "high." Many of these substances pass easily through the blood brain barrier.

Efficacy of the Agent

Some drugs are simply more potent than others in producing the desired effect. Each individual also seems to have a sensitivity to different drugs. Some can take or leave nicotine, while for others nicotine may be harder to stop than cocaine. Some opiate addicts have tried methamphetamine when they could not get opiates, and have come away hating how it made them feel, never wanting to use it again.

Stronger and more potent drug combinations are always under experimentation, to increase the speed and the intensity of the high. Probably one of the most potent reminders of this is the compound popular in Russia called krokodil, which causes immediate destruction of local tissue where the drug is injected, but results in an extremely intense high. The consequence is that people are losing limbs and body parts to tissue necrosis and gangrene, yet they persist in further use of the krokodil because the high is so intense.

Mixing drugs also can increase the intensity of the high. This is common with benzodiazepines and alcohol. The combination is much more potent. People try combining almost any combination of drugs to intensify the high, very often with extremely dangerous results. An example is pharming, which is growing in popularity among teens. Pharming is when the individuals at the party bring whatever prescriptions they can find, mix them in a big bowl, and take turns taking handfuls of the pills from the bowl. Anyone can see the potential disaster with taking multiple unknown drugs mixed together, yet teens perceive this as less dangerous because they think these drugs are actually safer since they are prescribed by a doctor.

IN THE ENVIRONMENT

Unfortunately, in our current society, there is nearly unlimited access to addictive substances or behaviors if we are looking for them. There is nearly unlimited exposure even if we are not looking for them.

Occupation

Certain occupations have higher risks, such as anesthesiologists who have ready access to the sedative and pain medications, or nurses who work in nursing facilities and spend much of their time passing out pain pills to patients who cannot report if they ever received them or not. Some occupations are more at risk for physical injury, or emotional and psychological stress, both of which increase the risk of taking or being prescribed addictive medications. Some law enforcement personnel not only have constant access to drugs, but at times they are even exposed to drugs while in the line of duty, such as undercover drug agents. Many other occupations have exposure to addictive substances or behaviors. Regardless of job or education, most workers are exposed to "social drinking," either during travel, after work as a way to relax, or during company parties.

Peer Group

During the teenage years our brains are still developing and trying to understand the relationship between our own behaviors and the consequences they bring. This is not fully developed until the mid-twenties. One desire we all understand early is social acceptance amongst our peers, but with undeveloped thought processes, teens fail to understand the consequences of the behaviors they adopt in order to gain that acceptance. Teens often feel misunderstood, undervalued, and insecure with who they really are and their peers have a huge impact on their sense of well-being.

In fact, we know from animal studies that social status and position do affect dopamine release, which explains the extreme influence of social pressures in our lives. Sadly, our society has adopted morals and behaviors which are incredibly unhealthy from physical, emotional and spiritual perspectives. Teens adopting these morals and behaviors, because they have become acceptable in society, are paying a heavy price. Involvement in sports teams has even become associated with an increased risk for drug use.

Teens who try to follow the Spirit of God often are mocked as outsiders and may fall away from their good choices even before they are fully capable of understanding the consequences of their decisions. It takes a spiritually mature and insightful youth to choose the guidance of the Holy Spirit over the physical and emotional rewards of social acceptance. Peer pressure still affects us as adults, and many of us simply adopt behaviors because our friends and family, or society as a whole, are accepting them as okay. Consider Las Vegas' recent motto, "What happens in Vegas stays in Vegas". Media provides a way for everyone to laugh at and then accept such previously unacceptable behaviors.

Culture

The tenets and traditions in a family have a clear and understandable impact. Immediate family culture has the most influence, as the children grow up with a basic set of life values. If these values reflect the teachings of Christ and emphasize being worthy of the guidance of the Spirit, then these kids are more capable of healthy self-guidance and avoidance of risky behaviors. If the family culture reflects the world's lack of moral values and acceptance of permissiveness, then we should not be surprised to see kids who experiment with all those things our society is adopting, such as pre-marital co-habitation, teenage sexual promiscuity, homosexuality, experimentation with drugs, social drinking, acceptance of violence and explicit sexuality in our media (movies, music, internet), and more. The list could go on and on. Our nation is adopting a moral standard of amorality. One of the biggest indicators of this is the demise of the family. Despite traditional Christian teachings, we are seeing men and boys becoming fathers without any commitment to their sexual partner, or the children which they helped create. The family is under attack, and is rapidly losing its standing as a Biblically-based model of a man, a woman, and their posterity.

Much more could be said about culture, but it should be clear how strongly cultural perspectives on addictive behaviors and substance use influence the risk of addiction. For example, cultural influences have at times expanded to encompass the globe. The drug culture of the 50's, 60's and 70's reached such proportion that an entire generation developed their own way of speaking, acting, and dressing. Many of the things we say now, the language we use, and some of the culture still around us reflects that era of time that grew in response to drugs, particularly marijuana and cocaine. Elvis, The Beatles, Woodstock, and many other names would immediately bring to mind the drug culture that existed during those decades, even if one did not live during that time.

Social Instability

Social instability has several potential meanings. As noted above, social instability can simply refer to the innate instability we are seeing in our society as the family unit is being destroyed. Without the family as the basic core of our society, we will lose the building blocks for moral grounding, and therefore lose unifying principles which keep this nation's people unified under God. We can never really achieve political stability when we stand on opposite sides of fundamental moral issues, for the term compromise has only come to mean, "move further to my side." If that side is Satan's realm of amorality, then any compromise only brings us closer to the pit. This alone will bring social instability as it leads to the collapse of a nation.

Additionally, social instability can refer to the social and economic status of individuals. Stress is a well-known cause of relapse, and also a factor in initiating substance abuse or instigating maladaptive behaviors. Poverty, terrible financial loss, and even an overabundance of wealth can all be stressors. Physical illness can be a stressor leading to social instability. Social environments filled with the maladaptive behaviors of others, such as gangs and cultures of drug use or physical and sexual abuse lead to social and emotional instability and stress. This, in turn, leads to a high risk of seeking an "escape" through getting high, or gambling, or finding "love" in a relationship that ends in the man leaving his "lover" and offspring as soon as the young girl finds out she is pregnant. It can mean finding "brotherhood" in a gang that often leads to violent death, jail, or an overdose on drugs.

IN THE HOST

Genetic Predisposition

We know that some individuals are more sensitive to becoming alcoholics than others. Research has detected genes (ADH1B and ALDH2) that are protective against alcoholism. Similarly, the gene P-450 2A6 appears to give some protective effect against nicotine addiction, as does P-450 2D6 against opiate addiction. Some genes also convey a higher risk of addiction. The gene CHRNA5/A3B4 increases nicotine dependence.[3] There is much to be learned in this field. This will help immensely in understanding addiction and finding treatments for addiction. It could also help us prevent addiction, by being able to avoid medications in certain people who are more susceptible to that addiction.

Multi-problem Families

Children's healthy development is highly dependent upon growing up in a safe environment. Many developmental studies have been done in the behavioral fields, observing both animals and children and the environment in which they are raised. Evidence is solid that healthy, loving and nurturing environments with a father and mother in the home, lead to children who have a better chance of becoming much more stable adults emotionally and socially, with less addiction and other problems. All families have problems of some sort. However, if parents do not have the tools to resolve crisis in a healthy way, the home stress builds. Then we add family moves (very common in our current society), with new schools and new friends. We add inevitable loss, such as death of loved ones, cherished pets, or loss of friends. In an unhealthy environment, these things can be devastating to a child's sense of security and well-being. In a healthy environment, they can actually build strength, teach appropriate grieving, and help build new bonds of love and security.

When divorce, drug abuse, or incarceration of a family member is added the stressors can become almost insurmountable to a child. Every little factor in an unhealthy environment can diminish a child's security and self-worth. If the family is not healthy and safe, there is no reason for the child to seek solace there, and they will go somewhere else. Studies of addiction have clearly shown a cascade of events, in which the more traumatic events occur to a child, the more likely that child will be involved with drugs and addictions. There are, of course, children from wonderful environments that make bad decisions, and children from terrible environments that make good decisions, but collectively, unstable family environments dramatically increase the risk of poor outcomes.

Co-morbid Psychiatric Disorders (Co-occurring Disorders)

Psychiatric illness has long been known to be closely associated with addiction. Substance abuse is closely tied to psychiatric disorders of all sorts. Often times those with mental illness are simply seeking a way to feel better or escape the devastation of the illness itself. We see many soldiers with post-traumatic stress disorder (PTSD) who become addicted. That is a commonly-known mental illness with associated drug abuse. However, many other illnesses have a similar impact on drug use.

There is also debate regarding the amount of impact drug use has on psychiatric disorders. Many drugs cause hallucinations, such as the young man who smoked marijuana and thought he was hearing God tell him to ride his bike on the freeway without holding the handlebars, singing with his iPod to songs which did not really exist. We know drug use can cause various changes and damage to the brain, depending on which drug it is.

In essence, we believe that psychiatric illness can make one more susceptible to addiction, and that addiction and drug abuse can cause or exacerbate psychiatric illness. This connection is commonly known as "dual diagnosis", or "co-occurring disorder", because of the distinct psychiatric component in addition to the addiction component, which are often seen together, and initially seem impossible to separate. I heard one speaker suggest that we should also talk about the "triple whammy", because addiction and psychiatric illness in combination almost invariably carry with them physiologic complications, such as liver cirrhosis, heart failure, abscess formation, brain damage, dementia, tissue necrosis, HIV, hepatitis, lung cancer, and more. This is a very valid concern, as we see the incredible costs rising from the complications of drug and behavioral addictions, not to mention the increasing toxicity of the drugs now hitting the streets.

SPIRITUAL SUSCEPTIBILITY

Another risk factor of addiction is our own incapacity for abstinence and/or moderation. Our spiritual capacity for good or evil often seems largely unknown to us as individuals. However, if we could each take a look back at who we were before we came here, I think we would be greatly strengthened in knowing our capacity is far greater than we think. We have been told this many times. We have been told that we are a choice generation, here to prepare for the coming of the Savior, worthy to live at the time when the Gospel has been restored in its fullness, to hold the Priesthood of God by proper authority. Alma Chapter 13 teaches us a little about foreordination and the priesthood. We have also been taught that we will not be tried beyond what we can bear. In his book Increase in Learning, Elder Bednar has told us this generation has a greater capacity for obedience than any previous generation. So, what is our spiritual capacity? What does that mean? How does who we were before we came to earth play out in our capacity to deal with addictions? This comes down to our capacity for obedience, for mastering our physical bodies, which when applied to the direction the Lord has already given us, means learning the value of abstinence and learning the importance of, and our capacity for, moderation in all things.

Many addictions can be prevented simply by abstinence. This is most applicable to things our body simply does not need, such as illicit drugs, which people choose to try for the sake of experimentation, popularity or many other reasons. This is applicable to any illicit drug of abuse, as it is to gambling, sexual behaviors before marriage and infidelity after marriage, and other things in which we simply have no need to participate. We have no need for nicotine, alcohol, methamphetamine, heroin, cocaine, gambling, pornography, or.... The list can go on and on with substances that are abused, and behaviors that lead to addictive habits of which we plainly have no need to ever partake.

However, it is not always so clear. There are times we will have exposure to things that are potentially addicting, which we must use with moderation. If we do so, we can safely use them. For example, using a barbiturate for seizures, or an opiate post-surgically for short-term pain management.

What about potentially addictive things to which we are exposed every day? What about food, and the epidemic of obesity? Sugar shows characteristics of being a potentially addictive substance. Yet we must have sugar to live, to create energy. What about sexual behaviors when, as teenagers, our bodies begin producing hormones and pheromones and other substances that drive us to sexual desires and behaviors? We must allow those natural feelings to be expressed to some degree in order to fulfill our purpose here on the earth.

In cases such as these, the answer is moderation. We need moderation for many reasons. Moderation can help us when we are careful and mindful of how much we eat, and what we eat. Moderation can help us with appropriate use of our natural passions and desires, not crossing boundaries of morality when we are dating, and then staying true to our spouse after marriage. Moderation can help us as we use pain medicine following a surgery, and then stopping it as soon as we no longer need it for the pain. Moderation can help us in managing the fragile balance between spending adequate time with our families, while honestly putting forth a full day's work for which we are paid, and dutifully fulfilling our callings in the church.

All of these important and good things can be unbalanced and lead to an unhealthy life. Certainly, we have all commented on the "work-a-holic" we have known. We have commiserated with leaders who spend so much time at church their children struggle, yet carry guilt for all the things they could not get done in their calling. On the other hand, we have seen those who completely neglect church, social, or work responsibilities, and never help because they are busy with "other things."

Any of these imbalances are potentially damaging to the individual and those around them. Again, these are not issues which we can judge externally. These are issues each individual must address with the Lord. Only personal obedience to the principles of the gospel, thus leading to the companionship and guidance of the Holy Ghost, can lead us to the answer in our own lives. The Lord will guide us and help us through feelings of happiness and peace (or conversely, feelings of frustration and discontentment if we need to change), to understand we are doing our best, and that is acceptable to Him.

It is so easy to become un-balanced in our attempts to live. We learn something, or become good at something, and allow it to become the most important thing to us. Moderation is so critical. We must learn to balance our lives. Not only can our weaknesses lead to our destruction, but our strengths may become just as dangerous. The following excerpt is taken from a talk by Elder Dallin H. Oaks, given at a BYU eighteen-stake fireside on June 7, 1992 in Provo, Utah; [4]

> "But weakness is not our only vulnerability. Satan can also attack us where we think we are strong—in the very areas where we are proud of our strengths. He will approach us through the greatest talents and spiritual gifts we possess. If we are not wary, Satan can cause our spiritual downfall by corrupting us through our strengths as well as by exploiting our weaknesses."

Elder Oaks then goes on to describe many areas of spiritual strength, and how they can be a danger to us. It is well worth reading as we consider our risk factors for addiction. I believe that pride in our own achievements, knowledge and professional prowess can become an addiction for us also. Elder Oaks ends his address with the following admonition:

> "How, then, do we prevent our strengths from becoming our downfall? The quality we must cultivate is humility. Humility is the great protector. Humility is the antidote against pride. Humility is the catalyst for all learning, especially spiritual things. Through the prophet Moroni, the Lord gave us this great insight into the role of humility: "I give unto men weakness that they may be humble; and my grace is sufficient for all men that humble themselves before me; for if they humble themselves before me, and have faith in me, then will I make weak things become strong unto them" (Ether 12:27).
>
> ...In all of this, we should remember and rely on the Lord's direction and promise: "Be thou humble; and the Lord thy God shall lead thee by the hand, and give thee answer to thy prayers (D&C 112:10)."

One of the most important concepts to glean from this chapter is that we are all at risk for addiction. Addiction has been fairly well defined, and traditionally we classify certain behaviors and chemical dependence issues as addiction. I would suggest that addiction is a very spiritual thing also. It has much to do with our spiritual-self being able to master and control our physical-self. If we do not do this, then we become slaves to all of those physical appetites and desires and passions, and thus slaves to Satan.

On the other hand, if we turn our lives over to the Savior and strive to follow the Holy Ghost, there is little which can enslave us. We must keep a balance, practice moderation, follow the Lord, learn humility, serve others, keep the commandments, develop charity, and love God and our fellowman. The scriptures are replete with direction of what we can do to have the Spirit in our lives. Prayer is our benchmark for following the Spirit, for as Mark Twain said through Huckleberry Finn, "You can't pray a lie—I found that out." [5] Honest communication with our Father in Heaven will set our hearts on the right path and guide us in the right choices.

CHAPTER 8

Repeated Use and Seeking Normalcy

"Through faith and righteousness all of the inequities, injuries, and pains of this life can be fully compensated for and made right... Through complete repentance of our sins we can be forgiven and we can enjoy eternal life. Thus, our suffering in this life can be as the refining fire, purifying us for a higher purpose. Heartaches can be healed, and we can come to the soul-satisfying joy and happiness beyond our dreams and expectations."

James E. Faust [1]

An unfortunate truth about the use of substances has to do with the development of tolerance. This is a defense mechanism of the body to protect itself against toxic substances, artificial physiologic states, and dangerous or hazardous demands on body performance capacities. However, this attempt to correct abnormal conditions leads to some of the long-term reinforcements for addiction. This chapter will help explain why addiction becomes such a difficult trap, as well as why it is possible to overcome.

Many addictions begin with recreational use of drugs in an attempt to escape, feel high, or just experiment. Some begin with legitimate efforts to control uncomfortable or painful conditions. Sometimes drug use begins for the purpose of enhancing performance, or just to make us feel better. Continuation of substance use often follows these patterns for a time, but then the substance use persists due to a desire to feel normal.

In trying to maintain homeostasis the body will use various methods of compensation to minimize the effects of the drug being used. In order to demonstrate this process we will consider the use of caffeine. Since caffeine is legal to use and readily available to everyone, most everyone has used caffeine in some form. Generally, it is in small doses, such as with coffee, or in soft drinks, or even in tablets to help stay alert while driving. Because of this, caffeine is a very good drug to use to explain how the body does compensate for repeated use of a substance foreign to the body. Some people are caffeine sensitive, in which case this will be a useful explanation. However, others have minimal effects from standard daily amounts of caffeine, which may make this a little harder to relate to the drugs which are more likely to cause tolerance and dependence.

Let us take an average person, who wakes up in the morning, tired, feeling less than fully rested, facing the tasks of the day. Or, the average person that by 3:00 PM is struggling to maintain focus and productivity at work or in school. All of us would love to have something to make us more alert, give us a little more energy to face the day, a little more productivity to push through tasks. All of us would like to have a little more focus as we try to complete the challenges that we face each day.

Caffeine has become an easy solution to these problems. Whether it be a cup of coffee or a caffeinated soft drink, we suddenly feel more capable, alert, focused, and feel exhilaration as well as accomplishment. We face our tasks and challenges with more energy and confidence.

However, often people who have positive effects from caffeine also develop a tolerance over time. After having caffeine on a regular basis, such as in coffee every morning, or a regular caffeinated beverage to help focus in college classes, that individual may find that they don't feel well and don't function well without their caffeine. This may be more true than they realize, as the body may compensate for the caffeine use.

Caffeine's effects are derived primarily by its impact upon the adenosine receptor, which is an inhibitory neurotransmitter. Adenosine makes us feel tired, sleepy, and fatigued. Caffeine blocks adenosine, thus directly countering the effects of adenosine upon our bodies and minds. Adenosine also blocks several other neurotransmitters that work in stimulating systems within the body, such as dopamine, serotonin, acetylcholine, and norepinephrine.

As a built-in safety gauge, adenosine protects us from over-stimulating and over-using our body. Adenosine helps remind us when we are overly fatigued, or need some time to recuperate and repair. Unlike a machine, our body is self-repairing and self-maintaining, as a general rule. It is generally not good to push for too long, or we run ourselves down, hampering our immune system, depressing our mood, and using up our reserves.

However, caffeine overrides those safety gauges, and lets us think we can push on even when the danger meter is running in the yellow. Some people count this as a wonderful thing, as they can function longer, and at higher levels. However, that effect is short term. Even so, most people think that because caffeine perks them up every time they use it, they are persisting with those long-term benefits, even though the body may be compensating for the caffeine use.

That individual may actually be only functioning at normal when caffeine is on board, and below normal without it. The body may have compensated to the degree that someone who does not use caffeine may now actually be functioning on the same level as the person using caffeine. This is a similar mechanism to other drugs, but much less extreme. By the definition used in this book, caffeine is not addictive. It may be habit forming, but use of caffeine does not result in the damaging changes we see with truly addictive drugs. To better understand true addiction we must consider much more potent drugs.

Let us take opiates (pain medicines, heroin, etc.) to expand on this example with caffeine. Opiates when taken in large doses can induce a massive release of dopamine within the brain. This is illustrated in Figure 1, which shows a normal state at the beginning, followed by the sudden upsurge after drug use that leads to a euphoria, or "high," indicated by a random numerical value of 100. The drug (an opiate in this case) depletes dopamine reserves, and once the opiate is no longer in the system the euphoria disappears and withdrawal beings. Eventually the body recovers, or compensates, and returns itself to a state of homeostasis.

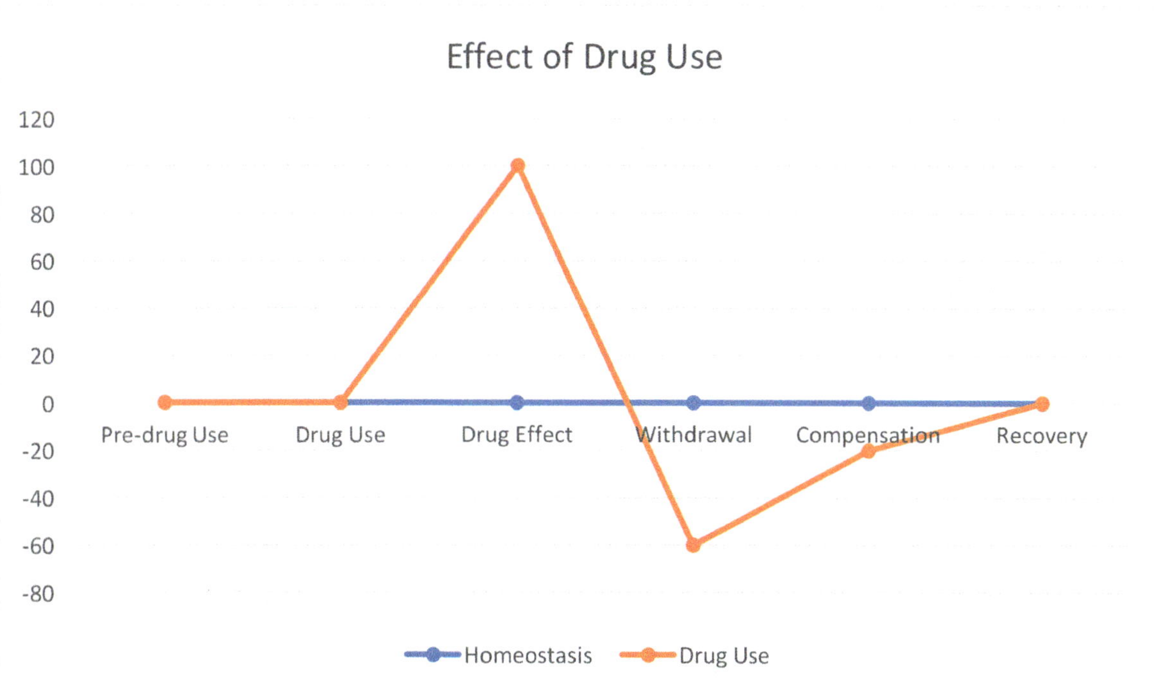

FIGURE 1: This is a simple representation of what the body does in response to a drug being administered in the body. (Numbers on the left represent an arbitrary scale, 0 = normal, (+) numbers indicate a feeling of wellbeing or + drug effect, (-) numbers indicate withdrawal or negative symptoms.) The blue line is the body's balance (homeostasis). It is indicative of both the levels of neurotransmitters, and the feeling of wellness (or euphoria) caused by that neurotransmitter. The orange represents the effects of the drug on neurotransmitters such as dopamine, followed by decreasing levels of the neurotransmitter, followed by the body re-establishing a normal balance. The duration of each phase depends on the strength and type of drug, and the rate at which the body removes the drug.

The person who used the opiate felt so good from the dopamine surge that they again want to use the drug. Repeated use results in similar effects, though they are very unlikely to generate the same degree of euphoria. Additionally, the body compensates just as it did in the caffeine example, but in this case the compensation is more dramatic and long-term. As a result, if the person continues to repeatedly use the opiate, over time the effects of the opiate on the body will diminish,

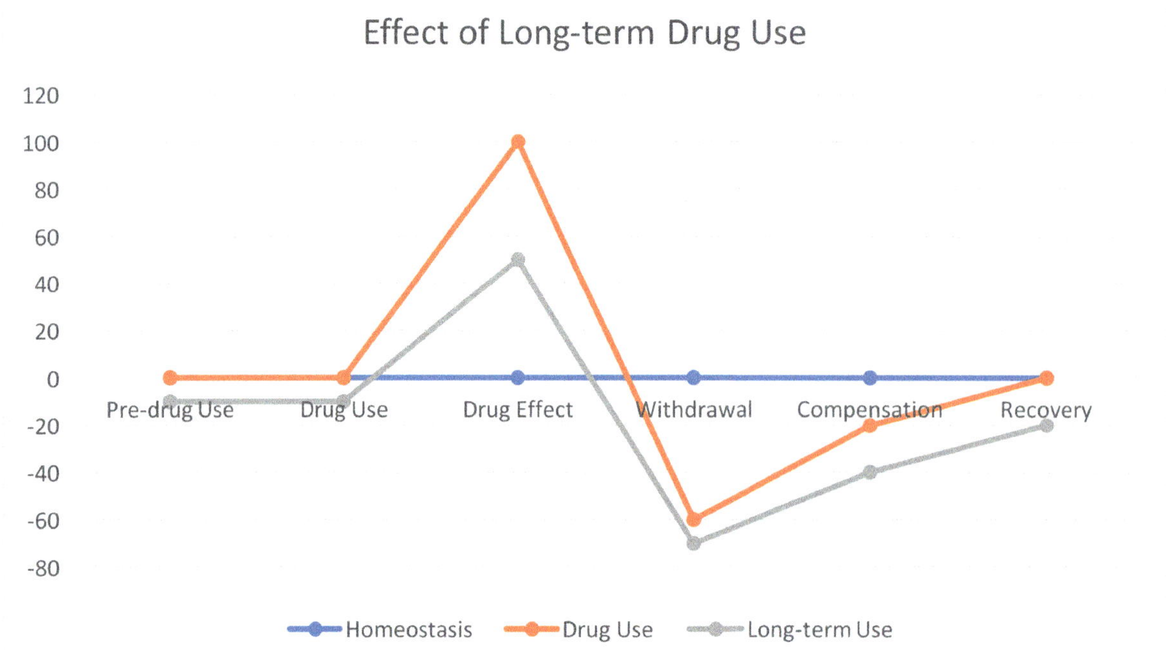

FIGURE 2: The gray line added to this graph represents the level of neurotransmitter in the body that develops after long term use of the drug. The body begins to lose the capability of returning to its normal level of homeostasis. Thus, only during the "high" does the person experience a feeling of returning to normal.

and less dopamine will be available, as illustrated in Figure 2. In this circumstance, the body does not fully recover, and the person's baseline wellbeing is now chronically below their previous state of normal.

Chronic drug use amplifies this problem even further, as depicted in Figure 3. The person eventually reaches the point where they have to use the drug just to feel normal. Without the drug in their system they decline rapidly into dysphoria, or withdrawal symptoms. After prolonged use, even when they do use, they often do not get high any more. Many times they use only to try and be functional and stay out of withdrawals. Many opiate addicts have told me they spend much of their time trying to find drugs simply to avoid the withdrawals, with little concern anymore for the high. Those that are still looking for the high switch to more potent drugs or try to mix drugs, driving the system further into disarray.

One of the complicating factors of this situation is that their brain tells them it can feel better,

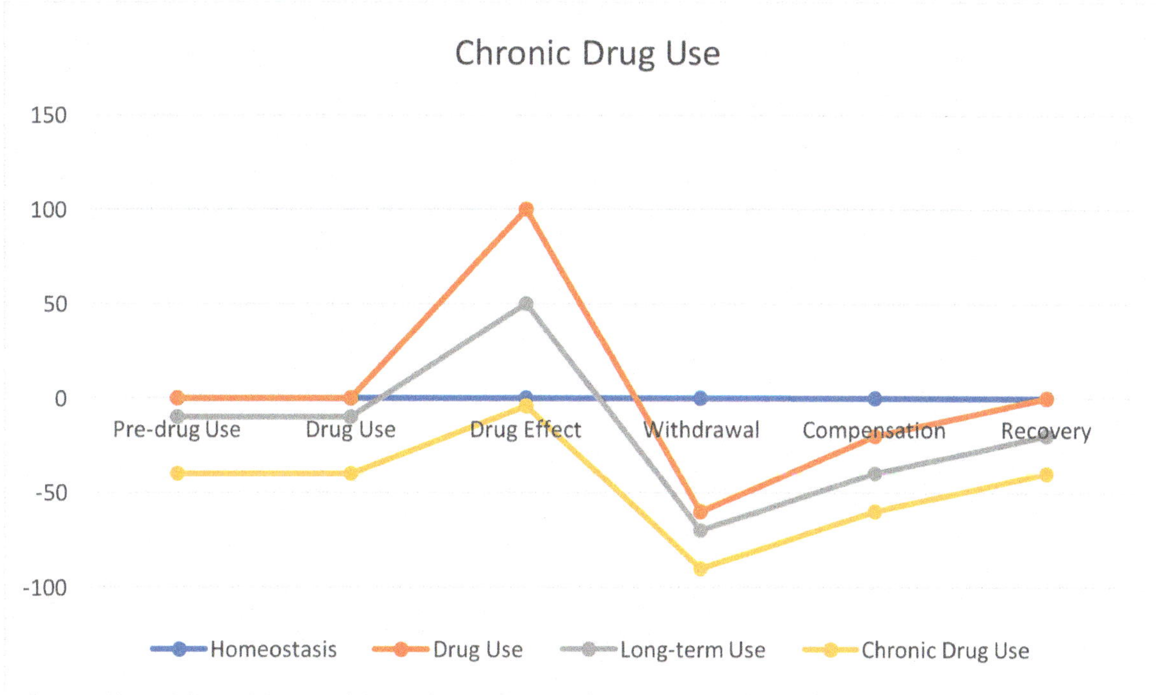

FIGURE 3: The yellow line added indicates the potential effects of chronic use. The body has compensated for the drug through various mechanisms, such that even with use of the drug one may only get back to the level of feeling "normal". This results in requiring a constant administration of the drug just to function day to day, hour to hour.

and they maintain a memory of how good they felt with their first "high." Many continue to seek that high, and are not content, even when they have drugs in their system making them feel normal. To them the normal has changed, and they want to always be back at that high. This drug memory (Figure 4) leaves them with an illusion that makes it very hard to treat because even after recovery they do not feel that normal is as good as it should be. To some degree individuals in recovery have to accept that they won't ever again feel that intense euphoria, and that can be very discouraging, and a very real risk for relapse. Using the drug again would temporarily restore a euphoria, but then it would rapidly shift back to the poor level of performance that was once experienced during the drug tolerant phase (Figure 3).

There are individuals who do not seek treatment and live every day trying to get along with a system which is compensating for the abuse. This is depicted in Figure 5. With many drugs it is possible to continue dosing the drug so frequently that the individual never goes into serious withdrawal. This requires having a constant supply of the drug in the body, and can maintain some stability, but it will still be generally below their original normal status. They will also be dealing with the drug memory that reminds them constantly that the drug should make them feel euphoric. Life becomes constantly painful and stressful for them. Their every waking thought is focused on the source of their next dose of the drug.

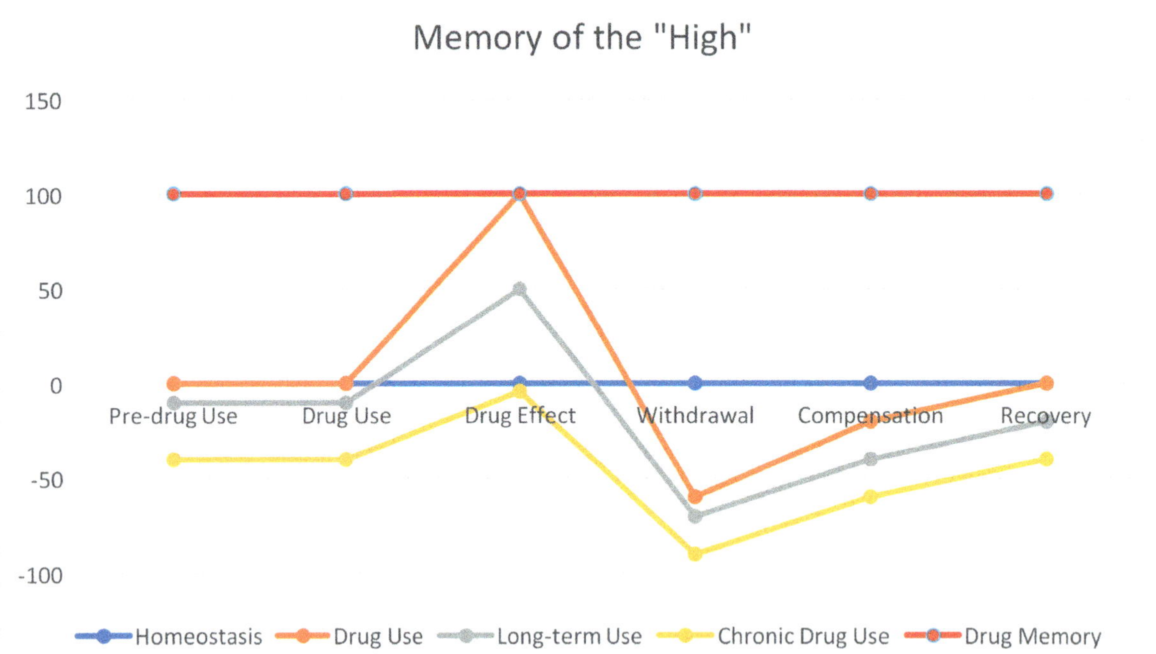

FIGURE 4: The red line added here depicts the brain's memory of the high—based on a chemically induced and artificial euphoria. Note how far above true normal this is, explaining the agonizing drive to once again get high. Also note how extremely far it is above the level of the chronic drug use, and how far below it the withdrawals can go. Is it any wonder that people use more and more, feeling so terrible that they will risk overdosing just to try and feel a little normal?

Happily, for most drugs of abuse the body can rebuild. Though it can be dangerous and uncomfortable, even to the point of the addict feeling they could die, over time the body may restore the natural neurotransmitters and rebuild the receptors. In other words, one can actually feel normal again (though not the new "euphoric" normal). It simply takes time. This is generally true of many drugs of abuse, though some of them can cause permanent and severe damage as a result of abuse. For example, prolonged alcohol use may permanently damage various organ systems.

Unlike caffeine, some drugs of abuse actually damage the body in such a way that physical, intellectual, and emotional healing from the abuse may not be fully possible. More and more of the street drugs are highly toxic. We unfortunately see many forms of damage by drugs such as methamphetamine, spice, and bath salts. Newer "designer drugs" seem to be developed with more carelessness and more toxicity, while searching for a substance that will produce a "better" high. Some systems in the body are irreversibly damaged, and the user will never again be the same.

The addict who now only uses the drug to avoid withdrawal is often the addict who finally seeks treatment. Of course, others may have legal problems, or the loss of everything important in their life that may drive them to treatment. Some have overdosed several times and literally believe if they do it again it will kill them the next time. These are examples of what they call "hitting rock bottom."

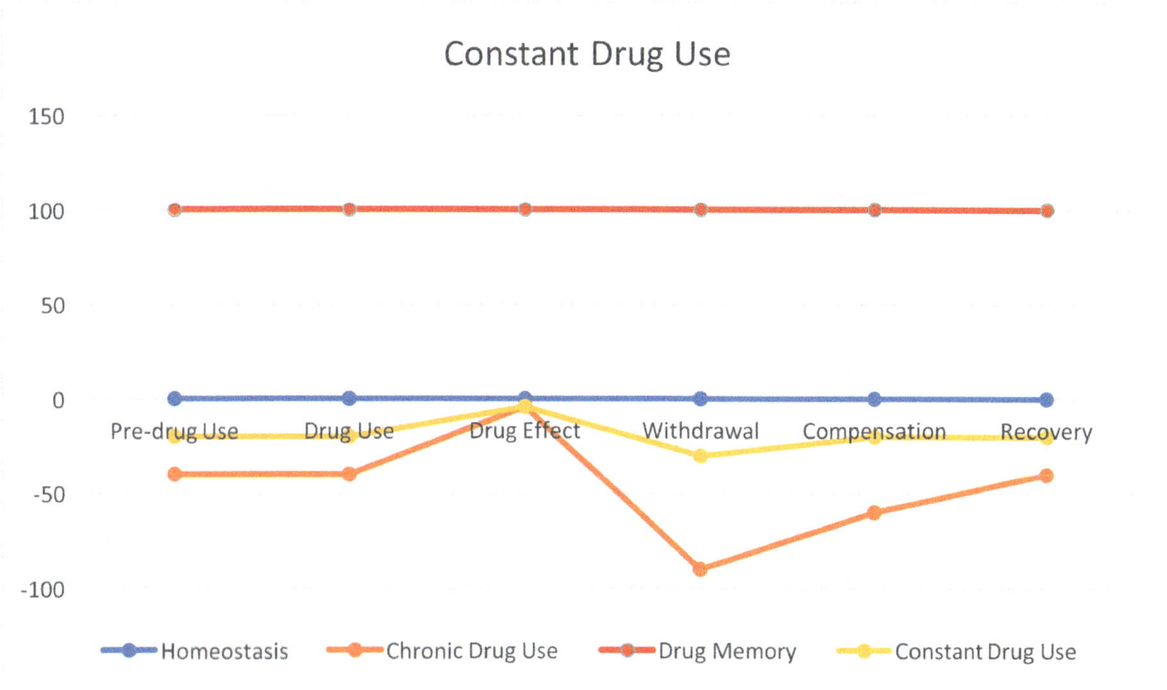

FIGURE 5: This figure is meant to depict the condition which develops in chronic use. The brain expects a normal of "100". Intermittent use produces lows as terrible as "-100". More frequent use of the drug minimizes the severity of the withdrawal, and helps maintain a more constant level of functioning—yet it is still below the level of normal body function, and far below what the brain perceives to be normal.

This is the point at which addicts finally realize the drug or their behavior is destroying them and they are ready for help. Before this, they have lived in the misconception that they do not have a problem, they can control their use, and they can stop anytime. Now, finally, they see they are at a dead end. At this point, they may seek the resources available to treat their addiction, and truly learn help is there for them.

A number of medications have been developed to avoid life-threatening withdrawals from addictions. Other drugs help with the discomfort of the non-life-threatening withdrawals and the control of ongoing cravings, to help prevent relapse. More medications are being developed.

Medications alone cannot treat an addiction, though. Many components of treatment must be added to build a complete program of recovery, including counseling, support groups, healthy living with a balanced diet and exercise, learning about addiction, along with supportive treatments such as massage, acupuncture, and most of all a faith in Christ. Whether it be the first attempt to attain recovery, or the battle back from a relapse, given the right tools, addiction can be treated.

SECTION 3

Addiction and the Gospel of Jesus Christ

CHAPTER 9

The Plague of Addiction

"Nevertheless, Zion shall escape if she observe to do all things whatsoever I have commanded her.

But if she observe not to do whatsoever I have commanded her, I will visit her according to all her works, with sore affliction, with pestilence, with plague, with sword, with vengeance, with devouring fire."

Doctrine and Covenants 97:25-26 [1]

A young man whom I had been treating for opiate addiction came to my office one day for his regular follow up. He was very nervous and quite upset. He had been doing well with his treatment, and had been "clean" from opiate use for nearly a year. However, he had recently relapsed. He told me that he had met back up with some of his old friends, and they had sold him some pills. His determination slipped, and he took the pills. Under my care he had been taking a medicine called buprenorphine, which partially blocks opiates (pain pills) from working. Because of this medicine the pills had no effect. He immediately realized he had wasted his money, and he also realized he had just experienced a serious set-back in his treatment plan.

As we talked about the circumstances of his relapse, I reminded him of something very important—those people were not his friends. They were anything but his friends. They did not care about his well-being or his sobriety or his ability to overcome a terribly destructive disease. In truth, all they cared about was his use and addiction to drugs so they could continue to make money from him. They did not care he could lose his job, his family, or even his life (except that he would no longer be their customer). As long as he was alive and struggling to feel okay they only cared that he would be addicted sufficiently so they could continue to squeeze cash out of him, to pay for their own drug habits and destructive life styles.

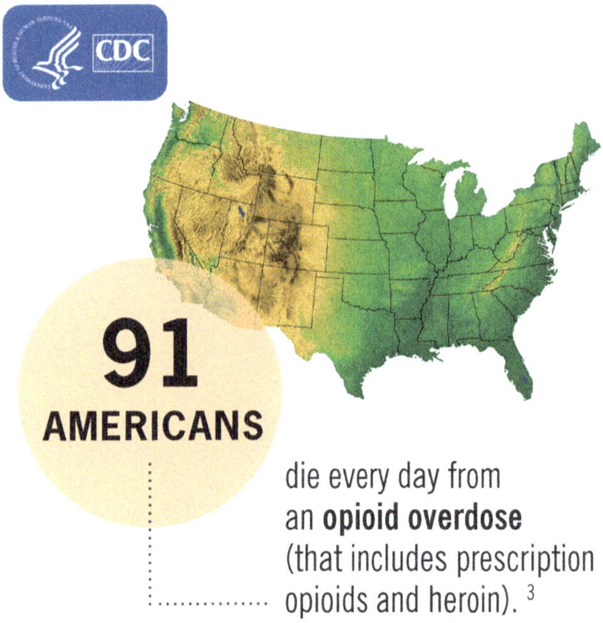

How much plainer can the Lord make it than to describe this situation as the "evils and designs which do and will exist in the hearts of conspiring men in the last days"?[2] We are no longer safe from these evils, no matter who we are. We cannot hide our head and hope they will pass us by, for they are everywhere. They are in the halls of our schools and on the playgrounds. They are in our homes, made popular on our televisions, and available through our computers. They are on the billboards as we drive down the freeway. They are on our cell phones and iPads. Satan has permeated every facet of our society, and successfully convinced us these things are okay. Our only protection is in listening to the Lord.

The Lord is aware of His children. He loves us and cares for us. He has warned us time after time of the troubles now threatening us, and of the trials which will beset us in the future. Often, He gives us very plain instruction to help us avoid the pitfalls that are so destructive, yet leaves us our agency to choose. But we either do not recognize the wolf waiting outside the door, or we think ourselves stronger and smarter than the wolf.

We all want to think we are strong. Yet, is it worth the risk to find out if we are really as strong as we think? Throughout the history of the world, there have been threats that have enslaved mankind. If it were not so, then ancient mariners would not have written about the lairs of the Sirens. Opium would never have devastated China, one of the greatest and oldest empires of this world. The prohibition of the sale, production and transportation of alcohol under the 18th Amendment to the Constitution in 1920 would not have led to widespread bootlegging. Men would not be ensnared by their indiscretions with harlots, or desire wealth or power beyond their needs. There are still those risks all about us if we allow ourselves to once enter into their grasp.

The Lord is aware of this. He did not leave us without warning and awareness. In our modern day, he has given us the following revelation:

> For I, the Almighty, have laid my hands upon the nations, to scourge them for their wickedness.
>
> And plagues shall go forth, and they shall not be taken from the earth until I have completed my work, which shall be cut short in righteousness—
>
> Until all shall know me, who remain, even from the least unto the greatest, and shall be filled with the knowledge of the Lord, and shall see eye to eye, and shall lift up their voice, and with the voice together sing this new song,...[4]

What does it mean, "and they shall not be taken from the earth until I have completed my work"? That work is "to bring to pass the immortality and eternal life of man."[5] What else besides personal righteousness through the Atonement of Christ shall bring that to pass? What if, in our day, we chose righteousness, never touching that unclean or forbidden thing? If we, as Christ's people, could do this, then perhaps the plagues would be lifted from us, and "cut short in righteousness." Perhaps we would learn to "see eye to eye" and "with the voice together sing this new song." Could this be the song we sing when we have only the desire to do the will of God, because we see it is the very best, most glorious, happiest, and greatest thing for us and those around us?

A man whom I shall call Mark came to my office with his wife, engulfed in the depths of his addiction. His wife was on the verge of divorcing him. He could not hold a job. He was in the throes of depression and anxiety. Mark was desperate. So was his wife. He truly wanted to change his life. Mark is of another faith, but he knew he had to trust in the Savior and give his life to Christ. In desperation, he came to see me, to help control his need for opiates. We discussed the options, and his wife made it clear that this was his last chance. Mark started treatment, and though he had some struggles, including relapsing several times, he has held to his path of recovery.

The key for Mark was he knew he had to depend on the Savior. Since our first meeting several years ago, Mark has made tremendous progress. His marriage is much better, though admittedly his wife still struggles at times with trusting him. Yet, as he sits in my office, I see the light in his eyes. He is happy. He has hope. He has not lapsed into episodes of despair and depression for a long time. He has not relapsed for several years. He rejoices that he is able to spend time with his grandchildren. Mark was very close to losing it all. In the end, he realized his family and his Savior are the most important things in his life. Mark is beginning to see "eye to eye" with the Savior. He is losing any desire to use destructive drugs. His desire to choose Satan's temptations is changing. He is beginning to "sing this new song" of righteousness.

Total American Deaths by War [6]

American Civil War	750,000 (420/day)
World War II	405,399 (297/day)
World War I	116,516 (279/day)
Current opiate overdose deaths	**(91/day)**
Korean War	36,516 (45/day)
Opioid overdose deaths from 1999–2015	**183,000 (31/day)***
Mexican American War	13,283 (29/day)
War of 1812	15,000 (15/day)
Vietnam	58,151 (11/day)
American Revolutionary War	25,000 (11/day)
Iraq/Afghanistan Wars* present	6,717 (1.57/day)
Philippine–American War	4,196 (3.8/day)

Consider the few civilizations that have lived in complete peace, and in the presence of God: The Nephites, after Christ's appearance to them; the people of the city of Enoch, when Christ dwelt in their midst; the people of King Melchizedek in

Salem. Perhaps there are other societies who have chosen righteousness, and chosen the better way. By their righteous desires Satan had no hold upon them. How sad that all too often we choose to give up our agency and allow Satan to chain us. When we fully utilize our agency as God intends for us, and become free through obedience and righteousness, Satan is chained, not us.

Addiction is certainly a plague in our day. Addictions of some sort impact every facet of our society, our communities, our jobs, and our families. It is rare to find someone who has not had a close friend or relative entangled in the webs of addiction. Our church leaders warn us ever more urgently and fervently of the rising dangers. They urge us to protect our families through teaching them the gospel and making our homes into sanctuaries where the Holy Spirit may dwell. The key is to have the Spirit with us, so that, as stated in verse 98 quoted above, we will "see eye to eye" with God.

CHAPTER 10

The Word of Wisdom

"Behold, verily, thus saith the Lord unto you: In consequence of evils and designs which do and will exist in the hearts of conspiring men in the last days, I have warned you, and forewarn you, by giving unto you this word of wisdom by revelation."

Doctrine and Covenants 89:4 [1]

There are many books written, and large amounts of data compiled from studies to analyze and interpret the principles taught in The Word of Wisdom. This chapter is not another attempt to analyze it or to interpret it, but instead is provided to reinforce the message it teaches us relative to avoiding addiction. This involves three key points:

1. The Word of Wisdom teaches principles that will prevent addiction.
2. The Word of Wisdom teaches principles of healthy living.
3. The Word of Wisdom teaches moderation

Prevention of Addiction

The Word of Wisdom contains a phrase that has puzzled me for years. In verse 3 we read, "Given for a principle with promise, adapted to the capacity of the weak and the weakest of all saints, who are or can be called saints." [2]

Why would the Lord say, "adapted to the capacity of the weak and the weakest of all saints"? I have wondered if the Word of Wisdom applies only to those who are weak. Who are the strong ones, and who are the weak ones? Is the Lord implying that all of us are weak? Some may be offended by this, and neglect obedience to The Word of Wisdom because they are sure they are not weak, and may choose disobedience to this law because they believe they are strong enough to overcome such things.

Understanding addiction may help us understand at least one reason for the Lord to say, "for the weak and the weakest," though there certainly may be many other meanings. The Word of Wisdom was given to save us from pain and suffering. In the final analysis, it does not matter who is weak or strong. Being mortal, we all have weaknesses. Our physical bodies bring weakness, regardless of our spiritual strength. Many of us have genetic predispositions to addiction. We do not know who that is, so in the end, if we follow the spirit of this law we can avoid even a potential addiction.

Even the "strongest" people are vulnerable when it comes to chemical and behavioral addictions if they allow themselves to be exposed to addictive substances or behaviors. The Lord has given us a way that we may simply avoid the potential for these addictions. Strict obedience to this commandment leads us to avoid ever trying alcohol or tobacco products. This is so important because none of us know where our potential for addiction may hide, and if we get caught in it we may become enslaved beyond our control to escape. Right now we do not know our genetic susceptibility without testing that addiction, which would be an incredibly dangerous way to discover if we are susceptible or not.

Certainly, there are circumstances which could expose us, even without making any bad decisions on our part, such as a doctor or dentist who overprescribes narcotics, or the family member who is trying to help a loved one who is in pain by giving them leftover narcotics. That is why it is so important to educate ourselves and others as to the risks of addiction. Then, if we begin to have problems, we know it is time to get help.

It is important to see the wisdom in this revelation. At the time it was given, the addictive substances discussed were quite common and accepted in society, being nicotine and alcohol. At the time, opium was available in various medicinal preparations, but there certainly was no methamphetamine, cocaine, bath salts, ecstasy, alprazolam, or heroin. The revelation simply warned us against wine or strong drink, tobacco, and hot drinks.

As we have gained knowledge of addiction we have learned much about the dangers of alcohol and tobacco. We are then able to extrapolate this warning in the Word of Wisdom to many other substances, such as methamphetamine, cocaine, heroin, ecstasy, and other drugs of abuse. In doing so it is not necessary to have further revelations regarding each substance. When we discover something to be addictive we can then take the wisdom given to us already, and avoid using any of those substances, just as we would alcohol and tobacco. It should be safe to say that anything which is potentially addictive should be avoided. Doing so would save us much pain and sorrow.

Hot drinks have been defined as tea and coffee. This can get very confusing at times. Many studies have been done showing potential benefits or potential harms with both teas and coffees. It is not clear why the revelation distinguishes hot drinks as not for the body or belly. However, just as they likely did not understand the concept of abstaining from strong drink and tobacco in Joseph Smith's day, perhaps the lesson to be learned is yet to come, and for now it remains to test our obedience. President Joseph Fielding Smith said, "If in doubt as to any food or drink, whether it is good or harmful, let it alone until you have learned the truth in regard to it."[3] It could be that these substances are addictive, or are simply harmful in some other way we don't understand.

Either way, this appears to be a test of faith and our willingness to be obedient even without a full understanding.

Most other drugs of abuse are quite clear in their effects upon our bodies. Of course, this is muddied for some people based on social and legal issues. Despite being legal, we know the dangers of alcohol and tobacco. We know they are both available and acceptable in our society. We also know that they dwarf all other drugs of abuse combined in terms of financial costs and health problems to our nation. Now we face the question of marijuana legalization. This is already beginning to cost our society in terms of social and financial implications, yet it is likely that the push to legalize it will be ever more successful in the coming years. There should be no doubt about marijuana, that it is an addictive substance (one of nine users will become addicted to it). There are potentially harmful effects as we now know, yet there are also potential medicinal properties that are being studied.

The debate over marijuana will be similar to many other debates regarding drugs and medicines. The Word of Wisdom tells us there are many herbs ordained for our use, and the Book of Mormon talks about the quality of herbs the Lord provided for the healing of various sicknesses. This topic, however, seems quite polarized. One side professes that only substances in their purely natural state should be used, and often even imply that if it is not natural, it is not safe, or if it is natural then it is inherently safe. The other side markets only products which have been purified and studied at length to determine the exact outcomes and side effects.

We must consider that some substances, such as foxglove, are highly toxic in their purely natural condition, whereas when a chemical from foxglove is isolated and purified it becomes a lifesaving medicine called digitalis. We must also consider that there are many herbs which are likely beneficial in medicinal ways. The difficulty is finding which of these herbs are truly effective and have any evidence to support their efficacy. Unfortunately, on both sides of the equation, there are likely individuals who seek to profit without regard to the benefit of the consumer.

This debate then leads us back to the discussion on substances such as marijuana (and similar discussions will come in the future with other drugs of abuse). While there are beneficial effects from using marijuana, they also come at high risk of detrimental effects. We would, in this case, do well to wait for further studies which can isolate and identify the helpful components in marijuana rather than consume everything in marijuana hoping for a small benefit which would be dwarfed by the ill effects of marijuana.

The Word of Wisdom has given us a model of avoidance for potentially addictive substances. It is relatively easy for us to draw from the direction given for alcohol and tobacco, and use the same wisdom in avoiding any substance of abuse. This is easy within the realm of drugs that have no medicinal value in humans, such as alcohol, tobacco, methamphetamine, cocaine, heroin, and others. It becomes more clouded in cases where there are medicinal benefit with medications that are potentially addictive, such as pain pills, sedatives, and mild stimulants. These substances fall more into the consideration of what the Word of Wisdom teaches us about moderation.

Healthy Living

The Word of Wisdom teaches us that there are many wholesome herbs provided for our benefit. We have been given herbs and fruits in their season. We have also been given meat and the flesh of beasts, as well as grains of all types for our use. It also appears when we read the instructions for these, we are to learn a lesson about moderation.

Herbs we have already discussed briefly. Anyone who has grown an herb garden has found great satisfaction in the delightful tastes of those herbs. It is likely, however, that the reference to herbs goes beyond making food delicious, and into the realm of medicinal benefits. Medications such as aspirin, digitalis, atropine, codeine, morphine, ephedrine, pseudoephedrine, quinine, scopolamine, theophylline, and vincristine are all plant derived. There are many more that have already been discovered and that are being used. There are likely many more which we do not yet understand, but which previous cultures may have understood and used.

When the revelation was given there was not medicine as we know it. Some medicines at the time were opiate derivatives and not well understood. Others were quite toxic and probably more dangerous than beneficial. With time, we have been able to find out why certain herbs are beneficial, study them, and glean the useful components from them. The Lord has blessed us with the science to do so, making them more available and more effective. It seems safe to interpret the direction given in the Word of Wisdom to mean herbs for both dietary (vegetables and spices) and medicinal purposes.

We are further instructed that the flesh of beasts and the fowls of the air have been given to us for our use. Again, we have polarization around these concepts. We have been told that these are for our benefit and use, but in moderation. However, we have proponents of veganism all the way over to those who propose that diets consisting of only animal proteins are the healthiest.

Our society is easily ensnared by the repetitious fascination with fad diets. Many of these diets actually work for rapidly losing weight—at least initially. However, long term data shows that nothing except lifestyle changes (healthy diet and exercise) will lead to effective and long-term weight loss. The real issue is that most of these "diets" do not encourage sound dietary principles. The Word of Wisdom is actually a very profound set of instructions on a healthy diet. Any diet undertaken should conform to the principles found within these few simple verses.

Studies on some of the leading causes of death in America (heart disease, cancers, strokes, diabetes) are fairly consistent in their recommendations: Our diet should be plant based, with less than 10% of calories coming from animal proteins, and based on grains, vegetables, and fruits. Unfortunately, our American diet is based on meat, fat, sugar, and starch. Herbs (vegetables and spices), fruits, and whole grains are considered sides and fillers, when they should be the basis of our diet.

The Word of Wisdom confirms this, that herbs and fruits are to be used in the season thereof. For most Americans, there is no longer a season, and we can enjoy the fruits and herbs year-round. In 1833 fruits and vegetables were only available in their season, or when they could be stored in a root cellar and preserved. Now we can enjoy them all the time without the risks of them being fermented or rotten.

Grains have been and still are available all year as they store easily, and we are told that grains are for our use. Our biggest mistake now is refining those grains and removing the fibrous components of the plants. Refining wheat into flour for white breads and pastas removes some benefits and increases the immediate sugar (one of the two potentially addictive foods) release in our body, which can exacerbate weight gain and other disease processes.

The consumption of various grains has been confounded by more recent health developments, such as celiac disease. This is an auto-immune disorder caused by the body forming anti-bodies against gluten, a component of several grains. When someone with celiac disease eats gluten containing foods, the antibodies attack the small absorptive structures in the small intestine, making that individual very ill, causing malabsorption, and increasing risk for gastrointestinal cancers. Gluten is present in wheat, barley, and rye. Unfortunately, this results in many people being intolerant to several of the grains. If they persist in eating those grains they can become extremely ill.

Celiac disease has been in the spotlight much more over the past two decades. Many substitutes have been found, and it is becoming easier to avoid the gluten. Oats and corn are still grains that are available (most people with celiac disease can tolerate oats if they are processed in a gluten free mill). The Word of Wisdom said all grains are good for man, even though it differentiates in verse 17 some preferences as to which grains man eats versus animals. One reason for this may be that the other grains (such as corn) are very good at helping animals (such as cows and pigs) grow and fatten quickly. Corn is also high in sugar content, and thus we have to be careful with diabetics. Wheat seems to be the most compact, the most easily stored, and a beneficial grain for man.

Meat is another controversial issue in our society, and in the church. Some are proponents of no meat whatsoever. Veganism goes so far as to avoid any animal product altogether. A careful reading of the Word of Wisdom teaches moderation, not abstinence. In the January 2013 New Era President Packer taught the following:

"Young people, learn to use moderation and common sense in matters of health and nutrition, and particularly in medication. Avoid being extreme or fanatical or becoming a faddist.

"For example, the Word of Wisdom counsels us to eat meat sparingly (see D&C 89:12). Lest someone become extreme, we are told in another revelation that 'whoso forbiddeth to [eat meat] is not ordained of God' (D&C 49:18)." [4]

I see wisdom in this as I watch people who have chosen to be vegetarian experience interesting results, including a lack of energy, the inability to stay warm, and difficulty obtaining all the needed amino acids a human body needs to stay healthy. Granted, in our day we are able to find complete proteins from plant-based sources. Yet, if one does not diligently work to maintain a complete protein diet, cutting out proteins can pose a health risk. The symptoms noted above may also explain why the revelation gives clear approval for using meat in time of winter, cold, or famine.

Research is telling us, however, that we use far too much meat in America. Some research data indicates that animal proteins should make up less than 10% of our caloric intake, and we should only eat 3 oz of meat a day (meaning all meals). Eating more than this likely contributes to heart disease, strokes, and some forms of cancer. Many experts agree that to prevent heart disease, strokes, and obesity we should not consume more than 30 grams of fat a day. Animal products are the primary source of our unhealthy fats. To put this in perspective, the average American consumes 85 grams of fat a day, and a piece of pizza or a hot dog contain about 13 grams of fat. A tablespoon of butter (or any oil or fat) contains about 12 grams of fat. Those food choices rapidly put us beyond the recommended 30 grams of fat a day.

Moderation

The United States is currently facing an obesity epidemic. Tremendous resources are being poured into the study of and the treatment of obesity, as it is being found to contribute to many of the more lethal chronic diseases we currently battle in America. What is being discovered is that affluent societies (such as America) are eating more, eating less healthy, and becoming more sedentary. The American culture also does not include as much of the healthier foods that other affluent nations eat. However, our biggest downfall seems to be our love of fat, sugar, and sitting around.

Certainly, genetics play a role. We do know that there are genes which predispose individuals to obesity. We also know there are complex physiologic processes, such as the interrelationship between leptin and insulin, that can cause weight gain, and can even create addictive-like behaviors in people when it comes to eating. These are very important for us to understand. However, we also know that the core issues leading to obesity are: too many calories in, too little activity, and poor food choices. This all leads back to the concept of moderation.

With his permission, I share the story of a good friend of mine. He is 6' 7" and at one time in his life he weighed about three hundred and fifty pounds. Being so tall, and being a strong and active man we all just accepted, to some degree, that this was how he was always going to be. However, during the course of time he discovered his blood sugars were high. In absolute shock, he faced the reality that he was diabetic. This was probably partly genetic, but also very likely to be lifestyle and obesity related. He was determined to solve this problem. Recognizing his part in the process, he committed to the Lord to change his life. He asked for a priesthood blessing to heal him, and went forward with an intense program of diet and exercise which was carefully studied, planned, and adhered to. Over the course of a year his weight dropped to 230 pounds (a very slim weight for a man 6' 7" tall), and his blood sugars returned to normal. We, in the medical field, call him a diet and lifestyle-controlled Type 2 Diabetic. He calls himself cured, through faith, a priesthood blessing, and a lot of hard work. He does not fool himself that this will not ever return, but he is aware of how to control it.

Yet if you ask him, he will tell you that he had to give up some things very dear to him. He felt he had to sacrifice a lot, particularly in the realm of the foods and the lifestyle he loved. He now also understands more about what an addict suffers in the behavioral components of addiction that are affected by dopamine. Though he never has had to deal with the physiological changes of introducing foreign chemicals into his body, he did have to deal with the physiological changes caused by years of being overweight. There were many. Bony structures actually changed. Physiological processes changed. His body is different than it would have been had he never become overweight.

Moderation becomes very important because there are many things in our lives that are potentially addictive, yet we must partake of them. This is where we truly learn to control the Natural Man and subject ourselves to the Spirit. We must, and should enjoy, participating in eating and sex. We need to be able to use medicines when we need them without abusing them. We need to have the joy and reinforcement from dopamine without letting it carry us to addiction.

In summary, the Word of Wisdom is a remarkable revelation which will help us avoid the trap of addiction. As addiction affects us mentally, emotionally, physically, spiritually, and financially, the Word of Wisdom is a gift given by a loving Father in Heaven to keep us safe and clean. With this in mind let us review the promises given at the end of the Word of Wisdom:

> "And all saints who remember to keep and do these sayings, walking in obedience to the commandments, shall receive health in their navel and marrow to their bones;
>
> And shall find wisdom and great treasures of knowledge, even hidden treasures;
>
> And shall run and not be weary, and shall walk and not faint. And I, the Lord, give unto them a promise, that the destroying angel shall pass by them, as the children of Israel, and not slay them. Amen." [5]

The 15 leading causes of death in 2013 were:

1. Diseases of heart (heart disease)
2. Malignant neoplasms (cancer)
3. Chronic lower respiratory diseases
4. Accidents (unintentional injuries)
5. Cerebrovascular diseases (stroke)
6. Alzheimer's disease
7. Diabetes mellitus (diabetes)
8. Influenza and pneumonia
9. Nephritis, nephrotic syndrome and nephrosis (kidney disease)
10. Intentional self-harm (suicide)
11. Septicemia
12. Chronic liver disease and cirrhosis
13. Essential hypertension and hypertensive renal dis ease (hypertension)
14. Parkinson's disease
15. Pneumonitis due to solids and liquids [6]

Certainly, this is not a promise of immortality. It is, however, a promise that we will be healthier and stronger than we would otherwise be, if we are obedient. It is also a promise connected to the rewards of eternal life, which are directly and eternally connected to obedience to living the laws of God. Obedience to God's laws qualify us for eternal life, at which point we will experience the fullness of all of these promises.

What about the meaning of finding wisdom, and great treasures of knowledge? Perhaps this means that we, through our personal application of God's law, will come to a personal knowledge of the doctrines behind that law. Looking at the world around us and what they suffer due to addictions, we already know we have been given great treasures of knowledge. Perhaps it refers to the things we learn when we attend the temple, worthy to do so. Perhaps we will come to a greater knowledge for ourselves that God lives, Christ sacrificed His life to atone for our sins, and that the Plan of Salvation is available to each one of us.

Joseph Smith said the key to salvation is knowledge. Wisdom is often described as the appropriate application of knowledge. How do we gain the greatest knowledge and wisdom? We gain them most quickly by being worthy to have the companionship of the Holy Spirit, for the Holy Spirit is our greatest teacher. The promises given in the Word of Wisdom are gifts granted to us through having the Holy Spirit as our companion and guide. The point of that promise is to help us understand that living the Word of Wisdom will help make us clean, and thus help us be worthy of that great gift promised to us at baptism: the constant companionship of the Holy Spirit.

This may be why we are asked about our compliance with the Word of Wisdom to determine our worthiness to attend the temple. The temple of God is the house of God. Where else could we hope to better gain that personal communication and guidance from the Holy Spirit than in the temple of God? In truth, we cannot expect to be taught effectively from on high if we are not worthy to have the Spirit to teach us, and we cannot truly expect to have the Spirit with us as completely as we are promised if we are enslaved to an appetite of our physical body, bound down by Satan's chains. Oh, the beauty of the Word of Wisdom in teaching us how to be free from Satan's grasp and how to enjoy more fully the companionship of the Holy Spirit!

CHAPTER 11

The Law of Chastity

"Because sexual intimacy is so sacred, the Lord requires self-control and purity before marriage as well as full fidelity after marriage."

Thomas S. Monson [1]

Sexuality is a great blessing given to us as part of the Plan of Salvation. It is wonderful, fun, exciting, rewarding, and can be the means of helping a couple bond with each other, in addition to their love, respect, and commitment to one another. Sex is also potentially addicting.

Though this book is focused primarily on chemical addictions, it is also intended to address gospel concepts related to addiction. Behavioral addictions such as sexual addictions follow reward pathways very similar to the chemical addictions. The primary pathway is dopamine-related, though it is also driven by hormones, and rewarded by adrenaline and other powerful neurologic responses. Because of this, the Law of Chastity must be addressed as one of the ways which the Lord has provided for us to help us avoid addiction.

Men and women have hormonal systems and other natural processes that cause them to be attracted to one another. These physical attractions are wonderful and God-given. They are to be enjoyed, and become part of a rich and full marital relationship. These feelings and attractions are also crucial if we are to fulfill our divine potential as God intended for us. Without these attractions, we would be less likely to obligate ourselves to the responsibilities of family and children. Perhaps we would fail to understand the importance of starting families, and likely even fail to understand the crucial role a family plays in God's Plan of Salvation. With society's decreasing emphasis on the spiritual meaning of families and more worldly acceptance of self-gratification, we are seeing the unfortunate results of sexual behaviors being used without self-responsibility or the acceptance of the consequences of those behaviors.

The physical drive for procreation will go ill for us if uncontrolled. That is why we are constantly being taught the importance of chastity and purity, in thought and deed. These teachings go on unchanged, despite societal fads and pressures, because there are very real and eternal consequences to sexual behaviors.The difficulty we face with immorality in our society begins at a young age, simply because immorality has become so commonplace, and is so readily accepted. We can hardly find a form of entertainment which does not portray some degree of immorality, and the world around us now expects us to accept it as normal, simply because they accept it. If we are not careful it may become too easy to express our dislike of such things, but then accept them as inevitable parts of our lives. In October 2003 Elder M. Russell Ballard instructed the church about choosing good media, and gave the following warning regarding wrong choices,

> "If we do not make good choices, the media can devastate our families and pull our children away from the narrow gospel path. In the virtual reality and the perceived reality of large and small screens, family-destructive viewpoints and behavior are regularly portrayed as pleasurable, as stylish, as exciting, and as normal. Often media's most devastating attacks on family are not direct or frontal or openly immoral. Intelligent evil is too cunning for that, knowing that most people still profess belief in family and in traditional values. Rather the attacks are subtle and amoral—issues of right and wrong don't even come up. Immorality and sexual innuendo are everywhere, causing some to believe that because everyone is doing it, it must be all right. This pernicious evil is not out in the street somewhere; it is coming right into our homes, right into the heart of our families." [2]

Elder Quinton L. Cook eloquently called for increased vigilance in our homes. With reference to the current discussion, one would benefit by a careful study of the entire talk. However, here I will only quote a short excerpt:

> "Parents must have the courage to filter or monitor internet access, television, movies, and music. Parents must also have the courage to say no, defend truth, and bear powerful testimony. Your children need to know that you have faith in the Savior, love your Heavenly Father, and sustain the leaders of the Church. Spiritual maturity must flourish in our homes. My hope is that no one will leave this conference without understanding that the moral issues of our day must be addressed in the family." [3]

Elder Cook goes on to relate his conversation with a young man who complained that while society at least recognizes the dangers of drugs, smoking, and alcohol, "there is no corresponding outcry or even a significant warning from society at large about pornography or immorality." Elder Cook then refers to a warning given by President Ezra Taft Benson: "We were warned at the beginning of this dispensation that sexual immorality would be perhaps the greatest challenge." [4]

If immorality in media is permitted in our homes then we eventually run the risk of accepting it. If we accept it we then accept the pleasurable response our body has to those stimuli. The dopamine begins to surge, the hormonal-driven desires go unchecked, and we lose control of one of the most powerful behavioral systems our God has given us. We are greatly affected by the hormonal changes leading to sexual desires and the body's chemical pathways that reinforce those feelings and behaviors.

Despite the pressures of society, I have seen amazing results with the youth who are simply taught correct principles. All too often we expect our youth to obey because they are taught the rules. Yet repeatedly, I have witnessed an amazing capacity in our youth to make good decisions if the doctrine is explained clearly to them. Once they understand the reason behind the rule they are much more inclined to live according to the doctrine, not just to obey a law. The pamphlet *For the Strength of Youth* was designed for the very purpose of helping our youth understand both the law and the doctrine. Often, I have heard the youth say, "I wish someone had just explained that to me before."

Our biggest danger is that what we have allowed our youth to see as "acceptable" or "unavoidable" in our society, is not pleasing to the Lord. Why? Because whether or not we think it is okay, or whether society thinks it is okay, if sexuality is depicted in any way except as a sacred, holy, and beautiful relationship allowed only between a husband and wife, legally and lawfully married, then it is not acceptable to the Lord.

Granted, there may be only one little tiny bad part in that movie (or book, magazine, game, etc.), but the rest is good and uplifting. However, that image, or thought, or seed of acceptance of inappropriate sexuality that is less than pure is in their (our) hearts, and only with great work can it now be removed to give way for the Holy Spirit. With less access and less exposure to the Spirit, our teenager (or ourself) thus has greater difficulty finding peace in their life and joy in their activities. Without the sweet peace of the Spirit, little seems to be satisfying, for truly nothing else will make us feel content and whole, and bring us peace, except the Spirit. Our youth then become irritable and unhappy. So do we. These exposures also trigger our dopamine reward system, reinforcing our desire for participation in immoral activities.

Indeed, without the Spirit readily in their life, they cannot find anything to make them happy, so they turn back to the one reward system that seemed to help them find some degree of pleasure: the ever-present and oh-so-powerful dopamine reward system that will give them pleasure in exchange for sexual behaviors, drug use, peer acceptance, and much more.

Hormonal surges seem to guide much of life as a teenager. This is good, and ordained of God, as long as these hormones lead to appropriate socialization, then dating, then courtship, then marriage. Yet we see in our society this process gone awry. Sexual gratification is sought without thought of commitment or the love that places someone else's happiness above our own.

Marriage, commitment, and families are thrown aside and replaced by self-gratifying sexual behaviors. The beautiful purpose of sexuality and intimacy are demeaned and lost in a world of pleasure-seeking to satisfy uncontrolled appetites. Because of our society's attitudes about sexuality, many people seek sexuality as the resolution to their problems, because society has so earnestly lied to us, teaching that sexual relationships are the ultimate end and most satisfying form of interpersonal relationships. While sex is certainly the most physically gratifying component of a relationship, it is absolutely not the crowning nor most fulfilling, defining, or lasting component of a true loving companionship. Sadly, society has forgotten we will never find lasting happiness in any relationship in the absence of the Spirit of God. In contrast, God's modern prophets and apostles have testified "that marriage between a man and a woman is ordained of God and that the family is central to the Creator's plan for the eternal destiny of His children." [5]

Let's look at how our youth may find themselves in harm's way. Take a righteous young man who feels a physical interest in a righteous young woman. Appropriate—if controlled. They think of each other, talk to each other, hold hands, and all the time experience physical, emotional, and even spiritual rewards for these behaviors, driven by dopamine and many other chemicals in their bodies, and (if their relationship is wholesome and appropriate) guided by the confirmation of the Holy Spirit. With self-control, the relationship progresses and appropriately blossoms into eternal covenants, with the priceless qualities of virtue, respect, and true love for one another, within the bonds of marriage where the appetites, thus far mastered, can now be experienced and enjoyed in a rewarding and fulfilling situation, bringing with them the blessing and companionship of the Holy Spirit, as well as potentially the wonderful blessings of children.

In contrast, consider the young couple that first indulges in talking, holding hands, kissing at an early age, and prematurely feeling the intense power of the rewarding behaviors of their body, with perhaps dozens of neurotransmitters and hormones involved before their minds and bodies are ready. It is not hard to see why they quickly deem everything else besides each other to be 'stupid' or 'boring.' As a result of chemical reinforcements, and instead of a true, respectful love in which appetites and passions are controlled, they give way to uncontrolled appetites.

Already, by stepping beyond the bounds God has defined as appropriate, these behaviors have become functions of stimulating the reward system rather than behaviors engendered by true love and true respect for the other person. They seek for escalation of the physical reward system, rather than the peace and joy that come with the companionship of the Holy Spirit to validate and reinforce a relationship and commitment to one another. To gain that physical reward, they engage in inappropriate touching and petting, and experience an even greater surge of dopamine and hormone-controlled behavioral rewards. Now, every time he holds her hand the big surge of dopamine no longer occurs, but he does experiences a small dopamine reward that draws his mind to the level of dopamine that he had with petting. They want that again. Holding hands just doesn't "do it" anymore.

Next time they are together, they discover that the petting and passionate kissing does not reward them as much as they expected, and the relationship progresses until they have sexual intercourse. This may result in bringing a child into the world, without a home where a father and mother have real respect for each other, much less are unified and committed to being a family.

Perhaps they will marry. Even then, they may find the dopamine reward is no longer as powerful as they once found it to be, and will continue to seek further means by which to achieve the same "high" that they once had. This is particularly true once the realities of family life, child-rearing, homemaking, and bill-paying settle in as more of a constant than the sexual intimacy which formerly consumed their every waking thoughts and had been the foundation of their relationship.

Dopamine release for doing laundry and going to work is generally insignificant compared to what it had been for sexual behaviors, particularly if these duties and obligations are not valued and rewarded within their relationship.

Pornography is a frequent escape for such reward seekers, more often for men. Women may find such rewards more commonly through lurid books and movies, which tell stories of secret passions and lust, forbidden loves, and escapes from the doldrums of everyday real life. These escapes become all the more enticing when one's own relationship is without the values of true love, respect, and eternal perspective. In people who are careless with their sexual urges, this is a process that often begins at a young age. It can, however, begin even after a person is happily married if there is indiscretion of thoughts and behaviors.

As the behavior persists, just as with other addictive behaviors, the reward lessens with each use. Soon other sources of reward are sought after, and extramarital relationships are pursued to satisfy those desires. The relationship that was held together by exciting pulses of intense neurotransmitter rewards and hormonal surges now lacks the deeper, stronger rewards possible from trust, love, respect, mutual interest and commitment that find their ultimate reward in the fruits of the Spirit—a reward far more powerful than that of dopamine or any other physical reward system. Lacking the excitement once thought to be the reward of the relationship, and not aware of any other satisfying reward to build upon, the relationship wilts. Marriages are broken, families splintered. This all starts so simply, yet so powerfully. Ultimately, this collapse is centered in selfishness, as the entire reward system was, in truth, a pursuit of personal lusts and self-gratifications.

In a general young women's meeting, Sister Elaine S. Dalton explained the following: "Your personal purity is one of your greatest sources of power. When you came to the earth, you were given the precious gift of a body. Your body is the instrument of your mind and a divine gift with which you exercise your agency. This is a gift that Satan was denied, and thus he directs nearly all of his attacks on your body. He wants you to disdain, misuse, and abuse your body. Immodesty, pornography, immorality, tattoos and piercings, drug abuse, and addictions of all kinds are all efforts to take possession of this precious gift—your body—and to make it difficult for you to exercise your agency." [6]

As a young married couple, my wife and I attended a marriage relationship class taught by the bishop. He taught a concept I found very powerful and very meaningful. He taught the only way a marriage relationship will truly thrive is when both parties have as their highest priority the happiness of their spouse. I will add one small key to his teaching: the happiness we must seek for our spouse is eternal and spiritual happiness. We will not succeed by striving for their worldly happiness. However, if we do everything we can do to make them happy and secure in this life, as well as every happiness relative to eternal covenants, at whatever cost to our self, our marriages will most likely succeed. However, our companion must grow in this also, and become more Christlike. Both parties must participate in the selflessness, and either one always has the freedom to choose otherwise. We cannot take away that agency. Both parties must act in the same unselfish way in order for any relationship to succeed. Amazingly, that concept flies in the face of physical appetites and our natural tendencies to protect ourselves, and therefore is the polar opposite of addictive behaviors, which are really just about "me."

So, what are the benefits of the Law of Chastity? First, it protects us from deeply painful and emotional mistakes, from which repentance can be very difficult, and full of sorrow. Lives are damaged when someone takes advantage of another person for sexual gratification, without any commitment. Unwanted pregnancies occur. Abortions are sought after. These are very emotionally devastating events, especially to the women who experience them. These can leave emotional scars and years of suffering.

Second, obeying the Law of Chastity through abstinence from sex before marriage also protects us from sexually transmitted diseases. If two virgins marry, there will never be a concern for sexually transmitted diseases. This is very significant as some sexually transmitted diseases are incurable, such as the Herpes Simplex Virus. Others can be deadly, such as the Human Immunodeficiency Virus (HIV), and Hepatitis A, B, and C. Moreover, a woman who is a virgin that marries a man who is a virgin will never contract cervical cancer, as cervical cancer is caused by the Human Papilloma Virus (HPV), which is a sexually transmitted disease. Unfortunately, sexual promiscuity is so rampant in our society that if a woman has ever had sex with more than one person, or has had sex with someone who has had more than one partner, we (as doctors) must assume that that individual has a sexually transmitted disease, one of the most likely of which is HPV, and the woman is routinely screened for cancer.

Third, disobedience to this law is one of the most destructive and devastating actions we can perform in this life. Through disregard to this law we bring children into the world without security, depriving them of the right of growing up under the safety and tutelage of two parents who are committed to each other and to their children. Sometimes they are left to wonder and learn from the world what is right and what is wrong. Disobedience to this law destroys marriages, and leaves children the victims of divorce and split families. Disregard of the Law of Chastity reflects the tragic misconception that marriage and fidelity and sexuality are subject to societal whim, rather than being one of the most sacred components of our eternal destiny and purpose. Neglect of this law wreaks its ruin upon generations to come until individuals find the strength and truth to redirect their path to be consistent with God's law.

Fourth, the Law of Chastity is one of the highest and most beautiful laws of the Gospel, bringing with it rewards of the Holy Spirit which we cannot gain in any other way, and which bring us nearer to God than in almost any other way we experience in mortality. Intimacy and sexuality are wonderful and essential components to marriage relationships. Creation and parenthood is a gift of Godhood which God has entrusted to us even during this mortal probation. In living the Law of Chastity, we get a taste of Eternity, mortal though we may be.

We know morphine is addicting. Morphine increases dopamine release by 200% of the normal. Sex does also. Morphine causes a more sustained release, but the intensity of the dopamine release is the same in both, providing a significant reinforcement for the person to want to participate in that activity again. This should make it very clear to us that sexual behaviors can be very addicting. Additionally, sexual desire is driven by hormones, social cues, and expectations, and many other components that do not drive one to use morphine. Sexuality is perhaps the most powerful naturally occurring drive in our lives.

The church has given very clear guidelines to help us learn how to control our sexual desires. Not dating before the age of sixteen, and going on group dates while young, are some examples of guidance given in *For the Strength of Youth*. The more closely we adhere to these guidelines, the more likely we are to avoid getting into addictive sexual behaviors. Once we are married we can then rightfully enjoy the blessings of sexuality with our spouse, as well as enjoy the blessings of the Holy Spirit in our lives, free from any bonds of addiction.

CHAPTER 12

Avoiding the Trap

"And finally, I cannot tell you all the things whereby ye may commit sin; for there are divers ways and means, even so many that I cannot number them. But this much I can tell you, that if ye do not watch yourselves, and your thoughts, and your words, and your deeds, and observe the commandments of God, and continue in the faith of what ye have heard concerning the coming of our Lord, even unto the end of your lives, ye must perish. And now, O man, remember, and perish not."

Mosiah 4:29-30 [1]

Having examined the impact of neurotransmitters and reward systems on our behaviors and choices, let us look at how complicated this becomes when we add chemicals that not only trigger these reward systems, but cause actual changes to our body's chemical and physical balance.

One example to consider as we move forward with this discussion is that of methamphetamine. Over the past several years there have been attempts to educate the public as to the outcome of methamphetamine use, and how devastating it can be. Many different "faces of meth" have been presented, in which we see a young normal looking individual, and then a second photo taken two years or so later. In the second photo, we see an individual who is emaciated, with sores all over his face and body, hair falling out, gaunt in appearance, etc. What is not explained is why this happens.

Methamphetamine stimulates dopamine release (and other reward systems) so far in excess of normal reward systems that the body's only desire is to gain access to more dopamine. In other words, the dopamine "pay-off" for using meth far exceeds the rewards for eating, for sleeping, for sexual behaviors, and all the other normal processes of life. Soon there is nothing else in life that brings any reward. A meth addict often quits eating because food simply does not provide a reward big enough to encourage the repeated behavior of eating when compared to the dopamine release caused by methamphetamine, or the devastation of the withdrawal that follows it. Meth addicts often freely engage in sex in exchange for meth, with little emotional or physiologic reward from participating in that behavior. Some would dispute this and say certain drugs greatly enhance the rewards of sex, but even that is eventually "burned out".

To make it worse, without the meth, the body experiences a severe dopamine deprivation. The only way to come close to understanding this is to imagine the very best thing you could ever experience, or even the collection of all the good experiences you have each day, and then accept that you can never again experience any of them, and there is nothing else in life that will ever bring happiness, or comfort, or contentment—ever again. That begins to describe how it feels for a meth addict to face the prospect of never having meth again.

The strength of methamphetamine addiction is frightening, but depending on an individual's genetic susceptibility, other drugs can be just as powerful, from marijuana, to nicotine, to heroin, to hydrocodone, to alcohol. The new "designer drugs" seem to be tapping into frighteningly powerful addictive potential, even while becoming more toxic.

One of the most tragic aspects of modern drug addiction is the practice of drug dealers to trap individuals in the addiction before they are aware of the dangers of the addictive substance. This assures the dealers a future market, and a lucrative one at that. The addict is enslaved even before he is aware that he has been trapped. This assures an ongoing flow of cash, or sexual servitude, or any number of other forms of dependent slavery.

We have seen, for example, the distribution of drugs such as ecstasy to elementary children, presenting it to them as if it were candy. The children then experience extreme physical rewards from what they thought was candy, rewards a child's mind should never be exposed to. It is well known the earlier an individual becomes addicted to a substance, the more difficult it is to recover from that addiction. This has been well understood in the arena of the "legal" drugs that are so frequently marketed in our media, and in the past, have specifically targeted the youth, such as nicotine and alcohol.

Research is showing that adolescent addictions meet with much higher rates of relapse, and have much less success in addiction treatment. Adolescent brains still have a significant amount of development that has to do with decision making and reward seeking. The capacity to understand outcomes of decisions and behaviors is developing until we are about twenty-three or twenty-four years old. Drugs can severely damage our capacity for understanding future outcomes. With early drug addiction, we often see adults who have never developed beyond a young teen level, emotionally and in their understanding of behavioral consequences.

Many times, we also see people using drugs because they just feel poorly, and their doctor gives them the drug because it helps them feel better. Unfortunately, as we have discussed, the prolonged use of many drugs simply makes the body feel poorly even though they are taking the drug. This is a common consequence with legitimate prescriptions of benzodiazepines for sleep and anxiety, and opiates for pain. I once attended a medical conference during which agents from the Drug Enforcement Agency (DEA) mentioned that the Mormons in Utah were really strong in avoiding alcohol and tobacco products, but someone forgot to teach them to avoid the opiates.

Some people say LDS people are just like anyone else, and because there is so much social stigma among Mormons about tobacco and alcohol use, they just find something to abuse that is more socially acceptable. Perhaps this is true, but I prefer (hope) to think this is more a consequence of ignorance as to the dangers of opiates and benzodiazepines. I believe many people begin using opiates innocently, and then find themselves trapped. I believe we, as saints, overly stigmatize addiction and are too fearful to ever admit we have a problem. Thus, we fear getting help. I even have disagreements repeatedly with health care professionals who do not believe that benzos and opiates are dangerous. If the health care provider giving the drug thinks it is safe, their patients would certainly have no reason to believe otherwise.

I also believe many who are addicted do not think they are addicted, or do not know that often times prolonged use of opiates creates or exacerbates their pain syndrome when there is really very minimal underlying pain (or perhaps no longer any pain at all). One of my greatest hopes in presenting this work is to teach the Saints in a non-judgmental way that opiates and other addictions are overpoweringly dangerous, but even so, there is hope of healing, feeling better, and being free of the opiates and other addictive substances. Nothing and no one is hopeless.

The simplest answer to the dilemma of addiction is to avoid addictive substances or behaviors altogether if possible, or manage them very carefully if they are a necessity for pain management or other legitimate purposes. Of course, we must be aware of the risks of addiction before we can completely avoid the traps. Education is critical for anyone to understand how devastating this can be. We must accept some people choose poorly despite their knowledge of risk. But rather looking on dispassionately as people wallow in the despair of addiction or sin, we must have empathy and love for them. For all of us have done this at some point in our lives. If it were not so, then we could claim to be free of sin. Only One was completely free of sin.

As we have also discussed, some people assume they are stronger than the addiction, and can just "do it a little." I would again warn that no one is stronger than these addictions, and even if that were a possibility, how would we know to which addiction we are susceptible? Satan will bind us as quickly as he can once we bend even a little to his desire. As soon as we give up the tiniest piece of our agency we then become slaves to Satan in that thing. Something as simple as a little lie can bind us, for lies beget lies to cover the previous lies. Addictions and wrong behaviors are simply lies in action.

Learning about addiction is so important. Even individuals who become dependent to narcotics following legitimate use, such as after a surgery, would know how to avoid the trap if they understood the highly addictive potential of opiates. An understanding of what drugs are dangerous and why they are dangerous may help youth choose not to use them. Knowing the names, the paraphernalia, and the effects of drugs could help parents detect an early problem. Knowledge can make us free—in a very real sense.

More importantly, living the gospel of Jesus Christ is the key to staying safe. Certainly, even obedient people who are striving to live the gospel can become dependent on prescription medicine, so knowledge becomes a personal obligation. This, however, is not to say that all opiate use or all benzodiazepine use is evil. Some will take this book to mean that no one should ever use an opiate for pain, or a benzodiazepine for sedation, because it will inevitably lead to addiction. Not at all. I believe, just as with all other knowledge that has been revealed in this day, there is a place for these legitimately prescribed medications. Several, however, truly have no medicinal value whatsoever and should be completely shunned (such as heroin, cocaine, PCP), and even legitimately prescribed medications should never be used without the skilled guidance of a knowledgeable professional.

There are many other ways that we can allow our physical bodies to take us into danger outside of drugs and medications. There are other physical reward systems besides neurotransmitters which can drive us to destructive behaviors. As king Benjamin taught, "And finally, I cannot tell you all the things whereby ye may commit sin; for there are diverse ways and means, even so many that I cannot number them." [2]. However, we can name a few.

Hormonal appetites and desires often drive us to try behaviors that can lead to addictions, such as sexual drives. Our desire for social acceptance, our emotional drive to find meaning with our peers often leads to unwise behaviors. Adrenaline (epinephrine), which has both hormonal and neurotransmitter effects, frequently leads people to seek behaviors which will enhance or increase the "adrenaline rush." I have heard many people describe themselves as "adrenaline junkies."

Elder David A. Bednar teaches us the following:

> "Satan also strives to entice the sons and daughters of God to minimize the importance of their physical bodies. This particular type of attack is most subtle and diabolical. . . . For example, all of us can find enjoyment in a wide range of wholesome, entertaining, and engaging activities. But we diminish the importance of our bodies and jeopardize our physical well-being by going to unusual and dangerous extremes searching for ever-greater and more exhilarating adrenaline 'rush.' We may rationalize that surely nothing is wrong with such seemingly innocent exploits and adventures. However, putting at risk the very instrument God has given us to receive the learning experience of mortality—merely to pursue a thrill or some supposed fun, to bolster ego, or to gain acceptance—truly minimizes the importance of our physical bodies." [3].

Chasing after extremes in our physical experience is not only dangerous, and minimizes the wonderful gift of a physical body God has given us, but it also drives us away from the Spirit. The Spirit will not try to compete with our desire for loud and overwhelming physical experiences. The Spirit will also not dwell with us when we minimize God's wonderful gifts that He has given us. We will fail to learn those things the Spirit would teach us, because we have removed ourselves from the presence of the Spirit. Anytime we succumb to the carnal desires of the flesh we remove ourselves from spiritual learning. Yet if we control our appetites and passions, and use them within the bounds which God has given us, we can find great joy in the gift of our physical bodies, in the presence of the Holy Spirit.

No one can truly live the Gospel of Jesus Christ without attaining the knowledge that teaches us what the Gospel means, what the commandments are, and what it means to live them. We have been given so much guidance and knowledge that few of us need to risk becoming addicted if we have studied the teachings of the Savior. The Word of Wisdom teaches us the doctrine and gives us a very solid base upon which to build. Resources such as For the Strength of Youth give us specific details of how to live. The Proclamation on the Family provides a framework from which parents can model their home. Repeatedly, the general authorities warn us and teach us in conferences, in devotionals, and in magazines. The scriptures give us models and warnings regarding the dangers of disobedience and indiscretion.

However, even with the needed knowledge, to some degree we all choose to ignore that knowledge and live unwisely. This is where obedience is key. Absolute obedience to the teachings of the Savior is the only safe path to freedom, and the only path to true knowledge. To choose to obey the Word of Wisdom, to choose to live the same standards taught to our youth, to choose to get help if there is even a little concern about being addicted, is within all of our power. To choose to live these commandments is the only way by which we will see the fruits of those commandments, gain a witness from the Holy Ghost of their truthfulness, and go on to enjoy pure knowledge.

Any of us may find ourselves so deeply in sin that we feel helpless to stop. However, we can always choose to seek help from our priesthood leaders, our families, and qualified professionals. None of us ever need be hopelessly trapped. To feel that way is natural (for the Natural Man is an enemy to God), but it is not spiritual. To feel that way is to deny the hope provided by our Savior, and thus deny the Atonement of Jesus Christ. The trap, then, is two-fold. One is to choose, through ignorance or disobedience, not to follow the Savior in the first place. He has shown us a path whereby we might tread in complete safety. The second is to choose, through despair, or embarrassment, or hopelessness, not to seek the Savior and avail ourselves of the suffering, of the price that he already paid on our behalf. It is already done. Let us be wise, and accept His gift to us.

There is hope. There is healing. There is the potential for every one of us, at any phase of our lives, to either choose to continue on the Lord's straight and narrow path, or to reach out to the Savior and plead for His hand to guide us back to that path. None of us will be forsaken. All we have to do is to seek our Master's hand.

CHAPTER 13

Obedience and Service

"I have learned a truth that has been repeated so frequently in my life that I have come to know it as an absolute law. It defines the way obedience and service relate to the power of God. When we obey the commandments of the Lord and serve his children unselfishly, the natural consequence is power from God. Power to do more than we can do by ourselves. Our insights, our talents, our abilities are expanded, because we receive strength and power from the Lord. His power is a fundamental component to establishing a home filled with peace. As you center your home on the Savior it will naturally become a refuge, not only to your own family, but also to friends who live in more difficult circumstances."

Richard G. Scott [1]

Amidst all the appetites and rewards we experience in this physical body, the most powerful reward we can ever experience is to personally feel the love of our Savior, for ourselves individually. This, I expect, is both a spiritual and a physical experience. Ultimately, this is why the Atonement of Jesus Christ has the power to change anyone that will accept Christ into their lives, insofar as they truly experience and come to understand the Love of God. This is how we change – or, perhaps, why we change. Once we have felt that love personally, no other reward system can overpower it, unless we simply allow ourselves to forget what Christ's love feels like.

We see the lives of many who have experienced Christ's love such that they have been willing to give up all else in their lives for it. Examples of this abound in the scriptures. Abraham was willing to sacrifice his only son because of his love for God. Prophets such as Nephi, Alma, Mosiah, Mormon, and Moroni, amongst many others, repeatedly sacrificed and served while giving up their own cares and wants. These men so aligned their wills with their love for the Savior that they were promised a place in God's Kingdom. In our modern dispensation, we see many more such examples of loving sacrifice. We see men all around us who sacrifice for the Savior, but certainly all of us can look to and appreciate the love and sacrifices manifest in such men as Joseph Smith, Gordon B. Hinckley, Thomas S. Monson, and others.

I always loved to hear President Hinckley, President Packer, and other apostles stand up and proclaim their optimism for the future, and for the time in which we live, despite the wickedness and the tragedies of the world around us. I believe they are so optimistic for many reasons. They know the will of the Lord, and are close to the Spirit. They also know the Plan of Salvation, and understand the promise of Christ's atonement. Yet I believe one of the greatest reasons they live with such optimism is because they have given their lives to the Savior and to the service of their fellow men. I believe that they, through their devoted service and self-sacrifice, have come to feel and understand what charity means, what the True Love of Christ really is, both in their own lives through devotion and sanctification, and in watching the glorious changes in other's lives as those they serve turn to the Savior.

Any who suffer from addiction, depression, despair, loneliness, or hopelessness would be greatly blessed in their struggle if they would but turn to the Lord by devoting themselves to the service of others. As King Benjamin taught, "[W]hen ye are in the service of your fellow beings, ye are only in the service of your God." [2] God will lift us, lighten our load, and strengthen our spirit. As Elder Scott taught us, there is great power that is bestowed upon us through obedience and service. God will give us greater power to overcome Satan's chains. His bonds cannot hold us if we turn to the Savior. What greater way is there to turn to the Savior than to lose ourselves in service and obedience to our God?

I do not imply there is no need for medication or counseling or other methods for the treatment of depression and other mental and emotional illnesses. However, I do contend that every person who loses himself or herself in service will find a great burden lifted, and will find they walk with a lighter step through the trials of this life. Only through service can we truly come to understand what the Savior did for us, and begin to understand the great cost at which He sacrificed for our sakes. Only in service can we truly come to understand charity, and understand why Paul taught us, that though we as individuals may have many great gifts, yet though we have great gifts, "and have not charity, [we are] nothing." [3].

A YouTube video by a psychologist named Kelly McGonigal called "How to make stress your friend" [4] is very enlightening, and is a brilliant discussion of how service can impact our lives. She talks about how stress, through the release of oxytocin (a neurohormone) prompts us to seek social interactions and physical contact, makes us more empathetic, and moves us to be more compassionate and caring. If we respond in these ways, this also leads to anti-inflammatory responses, including regeneration and healing to our heart. Ultimately, when we reach out to others, to either seek help or provide help, we get more oxytocin and more healing. Stress, under the proper response actually will make us stronger and healthier. People who cared for others while under stress showed no stress-related increase in death rates, compared to a higher death rate in those who had stress but did not reach out in a healthy way. This, then, can help explain the physical component of how service can actually benefit our physical and emotional health.

When we truly understand this love, all the physical "needs" of life become secondary. Loss and sacrifice of the physical aspects of life become tolerable, because we continue on with the love of Christ in our lives, and that will sustain us through all. Eventually we can become even as Abraham, willing to sacrifice all, with the understanding that through the love of Christ we can bear all things. We become as the great patriarchs and prophets in the scriptures, who did not fear death, for they knew their salvation was assured, which was far more important than any physical suffering or sacrifice. I am reminded of Elder Russell M. Nelson who, when he found himself a passenger aboard a spiraling airliner doomed to crash, felt peace rather than fear and panic at his apparently-looming death. I think of Abinadi who gave his life willingly in the testimony of Christ. I think of Stephen, who died while beholding a vision of Christ standing on the right hand of God. These men found peace in their lives through the pure love of Christ.

One of the simplest ways to feel the Savior's love is through service. Service is one of the most powerful principles, and one of the simplest to implement, and therefore one of the greatest tools that any of us have for recovering from the ills of succumbing to the natural man. As we give of ourselves to others, we begin to love others, and we begin to understand what the Savior taught us regarding Christ-like love. We begin to understand charity, not as a process of giving someone money, or material goods, but as a way of living, by loving everyone as the Savior loved them. Service is one way of practicing and learning about charity. We all desperately need to develop charity. As Mormon taught:

> "Wherefore, my beloved brethren, if ye have not charity, ye are nothing, for charity never faileth. Wherefore, cleave unto charity, which is the greatest of all, for all things must fail—
>
> But charity is the pure love of Christ, and it endureth forever; and whoso is found possessed of it at the last day, it shall be well with him.
>
> Wherefore, my beloved brethren, pray unto the Father with all the energy of heart, that ye may be filled with this love, which he hath bestowed upon all who are true followers of his Son, Jesus Christ; that ye may become the sons of God; that when he shall appear we shall be like him, for we shall see him as he is; that we may have this hope; that we may be purified even as he is pure. Amen." [5]

Through service we come to experience personally, and help others to feel, the Love of Christ. This is one of the reasons that programs such as the 12 steps of AA have been so successful, because they guide those seeking help to turn their lives over to God, and then reach out to serve others.

On June 5, 1976, I sat eating a meal outside my grandmother's home next to the Snake River just north of Idaho Falls, Idaho, during a family reunion. I shall never forget when a member of the family came running out of the house and announced we all had to evacuate—the Teton Dam had just broken. Nor shall I ever forget the outpouring of love and service that showed forth in those affected communities over the following weeks and months. Those who were involved still remember the loss and hardship, but they also still remember and talk about the loving service following the disaster.

In November of 1981 I was awakened from a nap on a Sunday afternoon to be told the small airplane in which my father and my uncle had been traveling from Idaho Falls to Salt Lake City had disappeared. My mother, two brothers and I immediately boarded an airplane to fly from Atlanta, where we lived, to Salt Lake City so that we might help in the search efforts for the lost plane somewhere near Soda Springs, Idaho. Despite the emptiness and sorrow that was in us for five months until the airplane was found, we were buoyed up by the selfless sacrifice of so many of our friends and family. Relatives both well-known and little known came to our aid. Friends from Eastern Idaho and from the Lost River Valley where I had grown up arrived, spending days searching, using snowmobiles, four wheel drives, helicopters and airplanes to help us. An uncle brought us Thanksgiving dinner as we sat in a hotel in Idaho Falls, contemplating our next move, and then loaned us his four-wheel drive so we could navigate the roads into Gray's Lake, Idaho. A farmer and his wife (complete strangers to us) gave us their bunkhouse and their food as long as we chose to stay, which was nearly a week. Even after the elements forced us to return home to Georgia, now destitute and fatherless, friends and family sent money that sustained us until the airplane was found the next spring. In all of this, I saw an outpouring of love I could never otherwise have imagined. I look back now, knowing we were sheltered by the outstretched hand of the Savior, through the service of our brothers and sisters.

To bear one another's burdens (whatever the burdens may be) is to serve our Savior. To give love and support and encouragement—to embrace the addict, or the sinner, or the wounded, or the fatherless, or the widow—is to live like Christ lived. As sung by Fontine in the musical "Les Miserable," based on the novel by Victor Hugo, "To love another person is to see the face of God." Though those who served me and my family may not know it, I now see the face of God as I reflect on those difficult times. As I listened to the beautiful voice of our neighbor as her voice cracked and she could no longer sing during the memorial service in Lost River, held for my father after his body was finally found, I felt her love and the Savior's love. As I cried uncontrollably at the graveside service in Santaquin, Utah, while my cousin embraced me, I felt the arms of the Savior holding me.

As we serve those in need, we will come to love them, and they will come to love us. In this love, they will get a glimpse of the Savior's love that is open, and easy, and real. It is perhaps one of the simplest ways in which both parties can feel the love of the Savior, and in doing so, choose to follow Him, and turn their backs upon the appetites of the flesh. Service is truly a path by which our bodies can be tempered, a path that can lead our spirits to become masters of our souls.

I am often able to measure the progress of a recovering addict by this very attribute of service. Many times, I have worked with people who are just not comfortable going to group meetings, being in group settings, and talking about themselves. Some feel their addiction is triggered when they hear others talking about their past use. Some are aware of dealers that go to the meetings looking for victims, and do not want to risk being offered a 'hit' because they cannot yet say no.

Then, after a time, they become more comfortable with those environments. They start to have the strength to face those triggers, that adversity. Finally, I can see the individual is making great progress when they voice a desire to help other people who are facing the same struggles. They want to reach out. They have strength to share. They care for, and feel the plight of, those around them. They feel hope in Christ. They feel the Love of Christ. Charity is working in their soul, and as they help others they better understand Christ's love for them. Ultimately, they can come to understand who they are, and why Christ loves them enough that He died for them. That is a remarkable change from the years of feeling worthless, lost, unhappy, and unclean.

Likewise, many families have struggled for years, hoping to help a loved one who has an addiction. Yet we all must be careful we do not mistake service for enabling, or being codependent. Those topics fill books, and are really the realm for qualified counselors, to help us understand how to help the addicted person, rather than harming them when we think we are helping.

When we learn those skills, we can draw boundaries, help our loved ones be responsible, and face the consequences of their behavior, all the while loving them as the Savior would love them, as sons or daughters of God. In doing so, we aid the healing process. And though there may be relapses, we must, as President Monson has admonished, always offer a safe port from the storms. He did not say to let them live at home as adult addicts so that they can spend their rent money on drugs. He taught us to offer a safe port where they may always return if they choose to live the laws of the Gospel, where they can come for healing, and hope, and to feel the Spirit of the Lord.

As we do this we will, through tears and trials, be able to love them, support them and teach them. We must do that which will bring the Spirit of God into our lives, so they will always be able to feel that Spirit when they return, as did the prodigal son. As we love them, we to will come to understand why the Savior gave His life for all of us—for the sinner, for the addict, for the thief, for the saint. We will feel that Christ-like love, and grow in charity.

Elder Scott continued in his April 2013 General Conference address, "As you center your home on the Savior it will naturally become a refuge, not only to your own family, but also to friends who live in more difficult circumstances. They will be drawn to the serenity they feel there. Welcome such friends into your home. They will blossom in that Christ-centered environment. Become friends with your children's friends. Be a worthy example to them. One of the greatest blessings we can offer to the world is the power of a Christ-centered home, where the gospel is taught, covenants are kept, and love abounds." [6]

Yet how do we build such an environment of safety, of spirituality? How do we recover from the devastating effects of addiction? We are brought back again to Elder Scott's teaching about the law which he learned: "It [the law] defines the way obedience and service relate to the power of God. When we obey the commandments of the Lord and serve his children unselfishly, the natural consequence is power from God." [7] Obedience is key, not only to our happiness, but to our progression.

Many feel that commandments and laws bind us down and limit us. That is not the case. Obedience to law makes us free. However, sometimes obedience is difficult, and often we are accused of "blind obedience" by those who find it easier to ignore law. They cannot see that disobedience will bring sorrow, pain, suffering and bondage.

For many years I wondered how to gain knowledge of God and God's laws. I wanted to know for myself, to gain the pure knowledge rather than having to depend only upon faith. I prayed for knowledge, for a solid witness of the gospel, of the laws. I reasoned that if I really knew, it would then be easy to follow the law. I wanted my faith to jump to knowledge, yet I did not know how to do it. I feared I simply did not have enough faith. I doubted the depth of my faith, and wondered if I would ever have enough faith.

Then, while I was bishop, I discovered more about faith. I realized that I had a lot of faith. I had spent my life trying to live the gospel, study and learn, progress, and follow Christ. I looked around me and saw many people, striving each day to live the gospel and follow Christ. That is faith. Such living is a grand expression of great faith. I had misunderstood faith, and underestimated its expression and power. Faith is not only to move mountains or give healing blessings. Faith is to strive to live the gospel every day of our lives, one day at a time.

This was further confirmed to me as I listened to a talk by Elder Jeffrey R. Holland. He said, "When problems come and questions arise, do not start your quest for faith by saying how much you do not have, leading as it were with your 'unbelief.' That is like trying to stuff a turkey through the beak! Let me be clear on this point: I am not asking you to pretend to faith you do not have. I am asking you to be true to the faith you do have. . . . Furthermore, you have more faith than you think you do because of what the Book of Mormon calls 'the greatness of the evidences.' 'Ye shall know them by their fruits,' Jesus said, and the fruit of living the gospel is evident in the lives of Latter-Day Saints everywhere." [8]

I think I am beginning to understand the process a little better now. Faith is expressed by learning and living the commandments of God. Faith becomes knowledge by continuing to learn and live the commandments of God. The only way to gain that knowledge is to experience it, personally, as an expression of faith.

A pertinent example would be the Word of Wisdom. When I was young I was taught the Word of Wisdom. In my home, I was expected to live that law. I also believed it was right, so I chose to abide by it. With the loving support of good parents, siblings, church leaders, and friends, I did live the law. Over time I began to see the unfortunate consequences for those who chose to disobey the law. My faith increased, and without outside support I began to live the law simply because I had seen what could happen if I did not live it.

Then, through my education as a physician, I began to see the blessings and benefits of living the concepts of health taught by the Word of Wisdom. The Holy Ghost confirmed those truths to me as science presented them, and also gave me a deeper understanding of those truths than science alone could have done. I have seen much to support the teachings regarding foods and lifestyles that support the Word of Wisdom. In addition, I have seen the truth in the teachings about alcohol, hot drinks, and tobacco. I have learned, through personal and vivid experience, the truths taught in the Word of Wisdom. Now, after years of living the law, I can truly say that I have a knowledge—a real knowledge—about the law known as the Word of Wisdom. I no longer live it by faith. I live it because I know it is true. I also know that if I ever chose to turn my back upon that knowledge, I would suffer even as those have suffered that I am trying to help. If I ever did so, I might then lose that knowledge that I had once obtained regarding the truthfulness of the Word of Wisdom.

Obedience, then, is the key to turning faith into knowledge. We cannot expect to know any truth if we do not first test it. We cannot hope to know the ways of God and the character of God if we do not choose to be obedient to those laws given by God. The Apostle John tells us, "And this is life eternal, that they might know thee, the only true God, and Jesus Christ, whom thou has sent." [9]

Obedience is the stepping stone, and it is essential if we expect to learn truth. Faith leads to obedience. Obedience brings the Holy Ghost into our lives. The Holy Ghost bears witness to us, both through the feelings of the Spirit, and by the blessings in our lives that come from obedience to that law. The Holy Ghost then teaches us, bringing that knowledge of the truthfulness of the law.

As we learn of the truthfulness of the gospel of Jesus Christ and all other laws that He has given us, we learn, as the Apostle Peter taught, "that by these ye might be partakers of the divine nature, having escaped the corruption that is in the world through lust. And beside this, giving all diligence, add to your faith virtue, and to virtue knowledge; And to knowledge temperance; and to temperance patience; and to patience godliness; And to godliness brotherly kindness, and to brotherly kindness charity." [10]

Thus, Peter teaches us that diligence (enduring in obedience), faith, and virtue (in thoughts and actions), leads us to the characteristics and qualities of Jesus Christ and God the Father, culminating with charity. Thus, we can become like God, and be able to abide the presence of God. Reflect upon these teachings:

> "Let thy bowels also be full of charity towards all men, and to the household of faith, and let virtue garnish thy thoughts unceasingly; then shall thy confidence wax strong in the presence of God; and the doctrine of the priesthood shall distil upon thy soul as the dews from heaven.
>
> "The Holy Ghost shall be thy constant companion, and thy scepter an unchanging scepter of righteousness and truth; and thy dominion shall be an everlasting dominion, and without compulsory means it shall flow unto thee forever and ever." [11]

How blessed we would be to be able to stand with confidence in the presence of God, and to have truth and knowledge poured down upon us as the dews from heaven. How blessed we would be to have the Holy Ghost as our constant companion, for it is the Holy Ghost that seals our covenants into eternal blessings. By our righteousness and obedience, we seek to be justified, and through the Holy Ghost we are sanctified through the Atonement of Christ, overcoming our weaknesses and frailties, until we are perfected in Christ, and are blessed with Eternal Life.

Obedience, as we seek after the knowledge of God, for the purpose of becoming like God, leads us to the ultimate purpose of this mortality. Charity brings us to the capacity to be like Christ, to understand what Christ did for us. To know God and Christ. To be as God and Christ. This is our purpose.

In his book Increase in Learning, Elder David A. Bednar quotes Elder Neil A. Maxwell's teachings from a devotional at BYU Idaho in 1997. Elder Maxwell said, "The youth of this generation have a greater capacity for obedience than any previous generation." Elder Maxwell then went on to quote President George Q. Cannon: "God has reserved spirits for this dispensation who have the courage and determination to face the world, and all the powers of the evil one, visible and invisible, to proclaim the gospel and maintain the truth and establish and build up the Zion of our God fearless of all consequences. He has sent these spirits in this generation to lay the foundation of Zion never more to be overthrown, and to raise up a seed that will be righteous, and that will honor God, and honor Him supremely, and be obedient to Him under all circumstances." [12]

Every one of us can do it. Addicted or not, in bondage or free. Whatever our place or station in life, there is absolute equality in the Atonement of Jesus Christ. The most righteous man needs Christ's Atonement, for he cannot of himself return to be with God without the help of Christ. The most addicted or lost man needs Christ's Atonement, for he cannot of himself return to be with God without the help of Christ. Yet Christ has prepared the way that both men, through the miracle of faith, repentance, baptism, the Gift of the Holy Ghost, and enduring to the end in obedience to covenants, may return to the presence of God, with confidence, to be blessed with an everlasting dominion.

This is the truth of the Gospel of Jesus Christ. This is the beauty of the message of Salvation, to be carried forth to all the world. This is the source of true and complete healing, from all addictions, all pains, all bondage, all abuse, all suffering and sorrow. As God himself explained to Moses, "This is my work and my glory—to bring to pass the immortality and eternal life of man." [13]

CHAPTER 14

Revisiting the Atonement of Christ

"To be saved—or to gain salvation—means to be saved from physical and spiritual death. Because of the Resurrection of Jesus Christ, all people will be resurrected, and saved from physical death. People may also be saved from individual spiritual death through the Atonement of Jesus Christ, by their faith in Him, by living in obedience to the laws and ordinances of His gospel, and by serving Him."

Russell M. Nelson [1]

Recently a friend of mine, Mike Webb, sat in my living room at my invitation to share his story. With his permission, I share his story:

Mike grew up in a family where his parents drank, and often quite a lot. His father worked at an airport and was frequently sent home with the small bottles of alcoholic beverages sold during airplane flights. These sat around Mike's home in abundance, easily accessible to him. At fifteen years old, he decided surreptitiously to try some.

By the time Mike turned seventeen years old, alcohol had become a regular habit. He joined the military and began using other drugs, such as marijuana. Stationed in Europe, he had direct access to the heroin coming from Vietnam. He used it on a regular basis, while passing the military's drug tests and functioning normally during his years of military service. Before he came home he "detoxed" in the infirmary over a week-long stay.

Once home, Mike continued on as a "functional" addict. He did not feel he had a problem. He worked in construction, doing a quality job, while continuing to use the drugs. He married and over time had five children. However, his wife also lived in the world of drug abuse, and their rocky relationship eventually ended in separation, and finally divorce.

Over time, Mike learned how to cook methamphetamine. He began making meth in large amounts and supplying clients who appreciated his high-quality product. Mike felt good about this. To him, it seemed he was participating in a worthy endeavor. Drugs were a way of life to him, and he provided a good clean (unadulterated) supply to those who needed it to function every day, including policemen, teachers, and many other professionals.

Mike eventually had trouble with the law and they finally put him in jail for cooking meth. During the next several weeks, he decided to stop making drugs, but within days of being released, he was back in his lab, making more meth. Once again he was caught and thrown into jail. After more jail time, he was again released on bail. He hit the road and ran for 5 months, hiding from authorities. One day he found himself with a gun to his head, a bondsman telling him to come along quietly or he would be shot.

This time the jail sentence was long. Things had not been going well for Mike before his arrest. He had been having troubles when trying to cook his meth. He could not find ingredients, and the recipes that he had never had problems with before simply were not turning out right. It occurred to him that perhaps God was involved in his life after all, and the time had come to change his life.

In jail Mike found a Bible. He also attended church on Sundays. He felt the Spirit, and began to learn the teachings of Christ. He was advised to study the New Testament first, and then the Old Testament. He did so, having much time to study and ponder. Over time he began to feel the Spirit of the Lord moving him to change. He learned the doctrine of prayer and fasting, and began to fast to have the cravings for drugs taken from him. Repeatedly he fasted and prayed, that he might be free from the enslavement of the addictions. Finally, one day as he lay in his bunk, he felt the desire to use drugs and alcohol pulled from him, as if something physical had been removed from his body.

That new beginning for Mike didn't end his struggles, however. When Mike got out of jail he contacted his father-in-law and mother-in-law. He had nowhere to go, and they offered to let Mike stay the night. This turned into a two-year living arrangement, under contracts and strict rules, while he got a job, obeyed curfews, and worked on the process of getting back in a relationship with his children. Mike and his wife could not make things work out, but Mike did progress, and his youngest daughter was able to move in with him again for her senior year of high school.

During this time Mike was also introduced to The Church of Jesus Christ of Latter-day Saints. Mike had discovered so many things in the Bible that he felt were critical, such as prophets and apostles, but he could not find these in their entirety in any of the churches he had attended, until now. With this introduction, learning of the doctrines of the restored church, Mike desired to be baptized. He worked towards that end, and after the proper process he was baptized. In time Mike fell in love with a woman he met at a church single adult activity, and they were married in the temple.

The path has not been easy for Mike. He regrets the years of his life "wasted" using drugs. He feels in some ways he lost the first forty-five years of his life. Now, however, he is actively involved in helping others with addiction recovery. He has been clean and sober for fifteen years. He is a devout Christian and strives every day to become a better person. He has no desire to use drugs or alcohol. He has come from what some people would consider an irreparable path of sin and sorrow, to being able to enjoy the most sacred covenants and blessings of the gospel of Jesus Christ. It has been a long and a hard road for Mike, yet Mike will tell you that he is a new man. Now he has hope, faith and purpose in his life.

Mike has been very involved in the recovery of others. He has actively participated in the Alcoholics Anonymous (AA) program through his years of sobriety. Over time AA has been one of the most successful ways to help people recover from addiction. Their 12-step recovery program has been instrumental in helping people come unto Christ. Any who have studied the 12 steps should not be surprised by the success of the program. Its principles are very consistent with the doctrines of repentance, obedience and service taught by the Savior. The first principles of the gospel are faith and repentance. The twelve steps first require that we acknowledge a higher power, which to us means God, or the Godhead. The steps of repentance (recognition, feeling remorse, making restitution, seeking forgiveness, and abstaining from the sin) are all addressed within the twelve steps. Then we must be prepared for a spiritual awakening, followed by the determination to be obedient to whatever God directs us to do, which inevitably includes serving others. Because of this consistency with the teachings of the Gospel of Christ, the church has adopted the 12-step model, with a few doctrinally-specific modifications. Step 12 is specifically all about service.

Throughout my career, I have heard much debate and been asked many questions about what specific model of treatment is most successful. There are outpatient treatment programs, residential treatment programs (which include twenty-eight day, sixty day, ninety day, one year, two year programs, safe houses, and more). We certainly do know that it can take years to allow the physiology of the brain and body and spirit to repair what can be repaired. We also know some of the most successful treatment programs have been the professional programs designed for pilots, health care professionals, and lawyers. These programs tend to be longer programs. The success of these programs, however, appears related more to the fact those professionals are engaged long-term simply by the leverage of maintaining their licenses and ability to practice their profession. For example, if a physician is engaged in treatment he or she is required to have consistent follow up for several years. If the physician does not do so then he or she loses their license and can no longer practice medicine. Thus, the consequences become leverage to continue treatment, and the longer someone is engaged in treatment the more successful will be the outcome.

Addiction treatment is primarily behavioral. The medical component can be a great benefit and a wonderful tool to aid in the detoxification and stabilization of physiologic processes within the brain and body. However, the behavioral treatment and the spiritual healing are key to recovery and sobriety. I have been asked by concerned family members what programs they should be looking for to help their loved ones. When they learn about the chronic nature of addiction the logical conclusion is the longer the program, the more successful the treatment. My answer is otherwise. The most critical component of treatment is the person with the addiction must simply begin the process of treatment, and be engaged in the treatment process. This can be done successfully in many different types of programs. That person will find many successful options if they are willing to engage. Factors to consider certainly involve cost (and whether or not cost or length of a program reflects quality is highly debatable), duration, and ability and desire to engage in treatment. Such engagement will necessarily involve a commitment to continue their treatment for the rest of their life. This may include participation in programs such as AA or other 12 step programs where the progression of healing involves helping others with the healing process. Ongoing healing also, of necessity, involves spiritual healing, which requires life-long spiritual maturation and growth.

My foremost hope, sitting in that restaurant in San Diego with my wife in 2004, was to teach of the Atonement of Jesus Christ. In doing so, I hope to teach that addicts can recover, they can be forgiven, and there is healing. Just as in the case with Mike, everyone has the capacity to change, and to come unto Christ. This applies not just to "addicts", but to all of us, equally. I have tried to provide some knowledge and tools to convince and persuade that such is the case, and to show a path by which this may be achieved. I have tried to show the vulnerability we all share, the danger of the natural man, and the power of obedience and service.

Ultimately, however, it is the Atonement of Jesus Christ that we must accept. As Nephi taught towards the end of his ministry, "And we talk of Christ, we rejoice in Christ, we preach of Christ, we prophesy of Christ, and we write according to our prophecies, that our children may know to what source they may look for a remission of their sins." [2] It is through Christ, and only through Christ, that we can be completely healed. We must be careful, however, that we do not assume we will be healed without effort, or simply by proclaiming our belief in the Savior. We also cannot expect that years of feeding our appetites and giving in to the natural man will quickly go away. It will take years to regain control and bridle those passions which we have unleashed. Addictions must be conquered one small piece at a time, one step at a time, just as they were created, bit by tiny bit.

Yet the glorious news of the Gospel is that it can be done! The Savior did atone for us. If we turn to him with full purpose of heart, he will strengthen us. Elder Bednar taught the following:

> "Brothers and sisters, it is possible for us to have clean hands but not have a pure heart. Please notice that both clean hands and a pure heart are required to ascend into the hill of the Lord and to stand in His holy place.
>
> "Let me suggest that hands are made clean through the process of putting off the natural man and by overcoming sin and the evil influences in our lives through the Savior's Atonement. Hearts are purified as we receive His strengthening power to do good and become better. All of our worthy desires and good works, as necessary as they are, can never produce clean hands and a pure heart. It is the Atonement of Jesus Christ that provides both a cleansing and redeeming power that helps us to overcome sin and a sanctifying and strengthening power that helps us to become better than we ever could by relying only upon our own strength. The infinite Atonement is for both the sinner and for the saint in each of us." [3].

Speaking to the missionaries at the Missionary Training Center in June 2002, Elder Jeffery R. Holland said the following:

> "...every truth that a missionary or member teaches is only an appendage to the central message of all time—that Jesus is the Christ, the Only Begotten Son of God, the Holy Messiah, the Promised One, the Savior and Redeemer of the world; that He alone burst the bands of death and triumphed over the captivity of hell; that no one of us could ever have those same blessings without His intervention in our behalf; and that there never shall be any 'other name given nor any other way nor means whereby salvation can come unto the children of men, [except] in and through the name of Christ, the Lord Omnipotent.'" [4].

In addition to this "central message of all time—that Jesus is the Christ," Elder Holland points out the beauty of the Father's gift to us, in sending his Son to die for us. He says, "The good news was that everyone's tomb could one day be empty, that everyone's soul could again be pure, that every child of God could again return to the Father who gave them life." [5]

We often hear outspoken people who are proponents of dismissing criminal charges related to drug use, or legalizing the use of certain drugs. Some of the reasons sound sensible; some do not. In our current political climate, we hear many say that legalizing drugs would lessen the health impact of drug use because they would not be so abused if they were legal. Some argue that legalizing drugs would decrease the cost to society because it would remove that expense from the criminal justice system. The arguments go on and on in favor of legalization, particularly in recent years regarding marijuana. Simply looking at the societal impact of alcohol and tobacco use (both legal, and both far costlier than the combination of all the illicit drugs combined) would convince any rational thinking person to realize legalization will not solve our problems.

I also frequently hear discussions related to needle and syringe programs, which have been shown to reduce the transmission of HIV and other blood-borne diseases such as hepatitis. These do seem to reduce the toll upon society by diminishing the impact of drug abuse. Similarly, treating opiate addiction with buprenorphine or naltrexone helps many people with addictions. But at what cost? In all of these situations, whether decriminalizing the use of addictive substances, or providing safe havens for treatment, we are expending a tremendous amount of resources trying to stop the ship from sinking, when we would have done better to prepare the ship before it left port. A wise philosopher said:

> "Society cannot exist unless a controlling power upon will and appetite be placed somewhere, and the less of it there is within, the more there is without. It is ordained in the eternal constitution of things that intemperate minds cannot be free. Their passions form their fetters."
> – Sir Edmund Burke

Any decision we make to disconnect ourselves from eternal law inevitably brings sorrow and suffering. As we let passions and appetites control our decision making, we indeed build our own fetters. We tie ourselves down with the bonds we have created through disobedience. In the Book of Mormon, the prophet Alma set out on a mission to the Zoramites. As an introduction to this mission, Mormon explains Alma's reasons for embarking on that mission. In verse 5 he states:

> "And now, as the preaching of the word had a great tendency to lead the people to do that which was just—yea, it had had more powerful effect upon the minds of the people than the sword or anything else, which had happened unto them—therefore Alma thought it was expedient that they should try the virtue of the word of God." [6]

Mormon and Alma are teaching us a very important principle: True change will not come because of how much we legislate, or punish, or educate, or provide social programs. The biggest impact will never come as a result of how much we threaten, or cajole, or work to fund programs with the intent of diminishing the social impact of diseases and drug use. One of the purposes of this book is to provide some knowledge relevant to the science of addiction. However, teaching about drugs and side effects and terrible outcomes is not the most effective method of preventing addiction. The primary purpose of this book is to show every person that the Gospel of Jesus Christ holds the key to solving these problems—even for the addict. The greatest thing we can ever do is to teach the Gospel of Jesus Christ! In 1943 President George Albert Smith (President of the Quorum of the Twelve Apostles) counseled the new Apostle, Ezra Taft Benson, "Your mission … is to … warn the people … in as kind a way as possible that repentance will be the only panacea for the ills of this world."[7]

We must teach faith, repentance and baptism. We must teach about the Atonement of Christ. We must help one another have a desire to live righteously so that we, as individuals and as families, have no desire to do evil. What a joy it would be to live as the Nephites did after Christ appeared to them, or as the people of the city of Salem, or the city of Enoch, and live together in a society where Satan is bound and has no power over the hearts of the children of men. What a blessing it would be to live with saints who understand the Atonement of Jesus Christ, the power of faith and repentance, who once having made a mistake know in whom they trust, and seek His Atonement in their lives.

Oh, that we could all share the heartfelt cries of Nephi, as he poured his heart into the record he made with his own hand upon gold plates. He left us with one of the scriptures' greatest expressions of love of the Savior and of His goodness:

> Rejoice, O my heart, and cry unto the Lord, and say: O Lord, I will praise thee forever; yea, my soul will rejoice in thee, my God, and the rock of my salvation.
>
> O Lord, wilt thou redeem my soul? Wilt thou deliver me out of the hands of mine enemies? Wilt thou make me that I may shake at the appearance of sin?
>
> May the gates of hell be shut continually before me, because that my heart is broken and my spirit is contrite! O Lord, wilt thou not shut the gates of thy righteousness before me, that I may walk in the path of the low valley, that I may be strict in the plain road!

> O Lord, wilt thou encircle me around in the robe of thy righteousness! O Lord, wilt thou make a way for mine escape before mine enemies! Wilt thou make my path straight before me! Wilt thou not place a stumbling block in my way—but that thou wouldst clear my way before me, and hedge not up my way, but the ways of mine enemy.
>
> O Lord, I have trusted in thee, and I will trust in thee forever. I will not put my trust in the arm of flesh; for I know that cursed is he that putteth his trust in the arm of flesh. Yea, cursed is he that putteth his trust in man or maketh flesh his arm.
>
> Yea, I know that God will give liberally to him that asketh. Yea, my God will give me, if I ask not amiss; therefore I will lift up my voice unto thee; yea, I will cry unto thee, my God, the rock of my righteousness. Behold, my voice shall forever ascend up unto thee, my rock and mine everlasting God. Amen." [8]

I believe there is nothing more powerful than the influence and the fruits of the Spirit. If we allow ourselves to bask in the love of God, manifest by the companionship of the Holy Ghost, felt as the Love of Christ, we will not need to depend on physical rewards. It may take a lifetime to learn this, to earn this, but when that day comes that we stand before God, if we have chosen Him and applied Christ's Atonement in our lives, we will know no greater joy and happiness.

No chemical, no behavior, no thrill of this world will come close to the reward of that joy, of standing worthily in God's presence, bathed in His love that we have learned to share with our brothers and sisters. As it says in the Doctrine and Covenants, "...then shall thy confidence wax strong in the presence of God." [9] Then we shall understand what true peace and joy and happiness are, and that they far exceed the realms of hormones, neurotransmitters, selfish sexual gratification, wealth, good food, power, or any other allure of the natural world.

Then we, as Nephi, will proclaim, "I will praise thee forever; yea, my soul will rejoice in thee, my God, and the rock of my salvation." [10]

References

Preface

1. 2 Nephi 25:26
2. https://www.cdc.gov/nchs/data/factsheets/factsheet_drug_poisoning.pdf
3. https://www.niaaa.nih.gov/alcohol-health/overview-alcohol-consumption/alcohol-facts-and-statistics
4. http://www.cdc.gov/nchs/data/nvsr/nvsr64/nvsr64_02.pdf
5. http://www.cdc.gov/nchs/fastats/accidental-injury.htm
6. https://www.niaaa.nih.gov/alcohol-health/overview-alcohol-consumption/alcohol-facts-and-statistics
7. https://www.cdc.gov/nchs/data/factsheets/factsheet_drug_poisoning.pdf

Chapter 1

1. Matthew 9:13
2. Timothy 1:15

Chapter 2

1. "Walk with Me," Henry B. Eyring, April 2017 General Priesthood Session
2. http://www.samhsa.gov/data/sites/default/files/NSDUH-FRR1-2014/NSDUH-FRR1-2014.pdf
3. https://www.samhsa.gov/data/sites/default/files/NSDUHresultsPDFWHTML2013/Web/NSDUHresults2013.pdf
4. Doctrine and Covenants 123:13–14
5. https://www.drugabuse.gov/publications/drugfacts/nationwide-trends
6. Doctrine and Covenants 121:45
7. 3 Nephi 9:12-13
8. M. Russell Ballard, "O That Cunning Plan of the Evil One," 2010 October General Conference

Chapter 3

1. Matthew 11:28
2. Mosiah 3:19
3. Discourses of Brigham Young, comp. John A. Widtsoe [Salt Lake City: Deseret Book Co., 1954], p. 70.
4. Jacob 2:17
5. Alma 41:11
6. Mosiah 2:17
7. Alma 22:18

Chapter 4

1. M. Russell Ballard, "O That Cunning Plan of the Evil One", October 2010, quoting audioenglish.net/dictionary/addiction.htm
2. Principles of Addiction Medicine, 4th Edition, 2009 by Lippincott Williams & Wilkins.
3. Center for Behavioral Statistics and Quality, National Survey on Drug Use and Health, April 7, 2011.

Chapter 5

1. "To Know God." Howard W. Hunter, 1974 October General Conference, Sunday morning session.
2. Adapted from: Di Chiari & Imperato, Proceedings of the National Academy of Sciences USA, 1988

Chapter 6

1. "O That Cunning Plan of the Evil One." M. Russell Ballard, 2010 October General Conference, Sunday afternoon session.
2. http://www.cdc.gov/nchs/data/nvsr/nvsr64/nvsr64_02.pdf
3. Principles of Addiction Medicine Essentials, 2011, pg. 20.
4. "Like a Broken Vessel." Jeffrey R. Holland, 2013 October General Conference, Saturday afternoon session.

Chapter 7

1. "Of the World or of the Kingdom?" Howard W. Hunter, 1973 October General Conference, Saturday morning session.
2. "Where Art Thou?" N. Eldon Tanner, 1971 October General Conference, Sunday morning session.
3. *Principles of Addiction Medicine*, 4th Edition, 2009 by Lippincott Williams & Wilkins.
4. "Our Strengths Can Become Our Downfall." Elder Dallin H. Oaks, given at a BYU eighteen-stake fireside on June 7, 1992 in Provo, Utah.
5. *The Adventures of Huckleberry Finn*, by Mark Twain, Aerie Books LTD, p. 213.

Chapter 8

1. "Woman, Why Weepest Thou?" James E. Faust, 1996 October General Conference, Sunday morning session.

Chapter 9

1. Doctrine and Covenants 97:25–26
2. Doctrine and Covenants 89:4
3. https://www.cdc.gov/drugoverdose/epidemic/index.html
4. Doctrine and Covenants 84:96
5. Moses 1:39
6. https://en.wikipedia.org/wiki/United_States_military_casualties_of_war

*https://www.cdc.gov/drugoverdose/data/overdose.html

Chapter 10

1. Doctrine and Covenants 89:4.
2. Doctrine and Covenants 89:3
3. The Word of Wisdom, *Improvement Era*, Feb 1956, p. 79
4. https://www.lds.org/new-era/2013/01/how-to-live-the-word-of-wisdom?lang=neg
5. http://www.cdc.gov/nchs/data/nvsr/nvsr64/nvsr64_02.pdf
7. Doctrine and Covenants 89:18–21.

Chapter 11

1. "Preparation Brings Blessings." Thomas S. Monson, 2010 General Conference Priesthood Session.
2. Elder Russell M. Ballard, "Let Our Voices Be Heard", October 2003 General Conference
3. "Can Ye Feel So Now," Quentin L. Cook, 2012 October General Conference
4. "Cleansing the Inner Vessel," *Ensign*, May 1986, 4.
5. The Family, A Proclamation to the World.
6. Elaine S. Dalton, April 2012, General Young Women Meeting.

Chapter 12

1. Mosiah 4:29-30
2. Mosiah 4:29
3. Increase in Learning, Deseret Book, 2011, p. 197.

Chapter 13

1. "For Peace at Home." Richard G. Scott, 2013 April General Conference.
2. Mosiah 2:17
3. 1 Corinthians 13:1
4. http://www.ted.com/talks/kelly_mcgonigal_how_to_make_stress_your_friend?language=en
5. Moroni 7:46-48
6. "For Peace at Home." Richard G. Scott, 2013 April General Conference.
7. "For Peace at Home." Richard G. Scott, 2013 April General Conference.
8. "Lord I Believe," Jeffrey R. Holland, 2013 April General Conference.
9. John 17:3
10. 2 Peter 1:3–7
11. Doctrine and Covenants 121:45–46
12. *Increase in Learning*, David A. Bednar, Deseret Book, 2011, p. 205.
13. Moses 1:39

Chapter 14

1. "Salvation and Exaltation." Russell M. Nelson, 2008 General Conference.
2. 2 Nephi 25:26
3. "Clean Hands and a Pure Heart," David A. Bednar, 2007 November General Conference.
4. https://www.lds.org/ensign/2001/03/missionary-work-and-the-atonement?lang=eng
5. https://www.lds.org/ensign/2001/03/missionary-work-and-the-atonement?lang=neg
6. Alma 31:5
7. George Albert Smith, in Sheri L. Dew, *Ezra Taft Benson: A Biography* (1987), 184.
8. 2 Nephi 4:30–35
9. Doctrine and Covenants 121:45
10. 2 Nephi 4:30

Additional resources available at:

www.lds.org

The Holy Bible, https://www.lds.org/scriptures/bible?lang=eng

The Book of Mormon, https://www.lds.org/scriptures/bofm?lang=eng

Doctrine and Covenants, https://www.lds.org/scriptures/dc-testament?lang=eng

Pearl of Great Price, https://www.lds.org/scriptures/pgp?lang=eng

General Conferences, https://www.lds.org/general-conference?lang=eng

Church Magazines, https://www.lds.org/magazines-and-manuals?lang=eng

For the Strength of Youth, https://www.lds.org/youth/for-the-strength-of-youth?lang=eng

The Family, A Proclamation to the World, https://www.lds.org/topics/family-proclamation

The Living Christ, https://www.lds.org/bc/content/shared/content/english/pdf/36035_000_25_livingchrist.pdf

Addiction Recovery Program, http://www.mormonchannel.org/listen/collection/addiction-recovery-program-audio

The 12 Steps* as Adapted by The Church of Jesus Christ of Latter-day Saints, http://www.mormonnewsroom.org/additional-resource/the-12-steps-as-adapted-by-the-church-of-jesus-christ-of-latter-day-saints

SECTION 4

APPENDIX

Introduction

Drugs which are abused come in many forms, and are available from many sources. The information contained in these appendices has come primarily from the National Institute of Drug Abuse data. Several other websites have been used and can be easily referenced on the following links:

- **Commonly abused street drugs:** www.drugabuse.gov/drugs-abuse/commonly-abused-drugs/commonly-abused-drugs-chart
- **Commonly abused prescription drugs:** www.drugabuse.gov/drugs-abuse/commonly-abused-drugs/commonly-abused-prescription-drugs-chart
- **DEA drug information site:** www.justice.gov/dea/druginfo/factsheets.shtml
- **Parents' resource site:** www.getsmartaboutdrugs.com
- **Foundation for a Drug-Free World site:** www.drugfreeworld.org
- **National Institute of Drug Abuse:** www.drugabuse.gov

When discussing drug use on a national or worldwide level, the numbers are astounding. "An estimated 149-271 million people used an illicit drug worldwide in 2009. ...These estimates probably underestimate the true burden..." [1] The numbers are likely much higher, as use is generally under-reported due to criminal penalties, societal stigma, insurance applications, legal licenses, and other many reasons which drive individuals away from self-reporting their drug habits.

Additionally, individuals with drug dependence often use more than one type of drug. Marijuana, alcohol, and tobacco are all commonly used drugs. Opiates are becoming very popular, and use tends to escalate through stages and potency to injectable forms such as heroin. Benzodiazepines and other sedative hypnotics produce a tolerance that requires escalation of doses. Such compounds also have the ability to enhance the effects of other drugs. New "designer drugs" are becoming more toxic and more addictive. Combinations of these various drugs lead to worse addictions, and an ever-growing strain on societal resources.

The human body wants to be in a state of balance called homeostasis. Using external substances to artificially stimulate our body's normal reward system leads to an imbalance in this homeostasis, and the body tries to correct itself. As a body's reward system is shoved into overdrive by external substances, the body then works to correct this response by diminishing the resources within the reward system to regain the natural controls of homeostasis. Users often add another drug to re-stimulate the reward system, chasing that first "high," or some other desired effect. Understanding the drug classes and their effects is key to understanding how the drugs affect our body's natural balance, how the body attempts to correct that, and why we lose our ability to feel good without the drugs.

The remaining appendices are primarily focused on a general explanation of drug classes and their effects, and other quick reference information. Though they are organized by drug class, keep in mind that combining any of these classes of drugs may make them more potent, more toxic, and often more addicting.

To make these reference sections more useful, they also include lists of chemical and trade names of drugs. These are primarily the drugs available in the United States, and are certainly not all inclusive. Many other drugs exist in each class throughout the world market. Information is constantly changing—new drugs coming out, new street names evolving, and new tactics for evading detection develop. Information floods the internet and it is hard to know what data is reliable and true. For this reason, I have included the links located above and at the end of the appendices as references for reliable web sites.

Overall, several issues are standard for any drug of abuse. Despite triggering different receptors and neurotransmitters, ultimately, they all compromise the body's natural reward system, and potentially damage the dopamine supply in the brain. Drugs of abuse also affect the areas of the brain having to do with executive function. In other words, they change our capacity to make good decisions, and remove inhibitions about dangerous behaviors, as well as making it more difficult to learn from bad consequences.

Much research is also underway regarding the body's glucocorticoid system, which is a system activated by stress. Glucocorticoids, when repeatedly or too heavily overstimulated, lead to a myriad of problems in the body, from mild symptoms of acute stress and anxiety to chronic diseases and organ system failures. All drugs of abuse activate these stress systems. Cortisol and other glucocorticoids released during stress are shown to play a role in addiction, as they do in many other illnesses, both physical and psychiatric.

As we discuss drugs in general, it is also worth noting in many cases people use drugs illicitly simply because the drugs help them feel better. It is very likely some people persist in using these drugs because they perceive a therapeutic benefit from them. For example, some people with Post Traumatic Stress Disorder, Schizophrenia, Depression, anxiety disorders, and other conditions do feel better (whether their symptoms are just masked, or actually controlled is hard to say) from the use of an illicit drug.

Therefore, it is very probable some individuals who use the illicit drugs do so because it is the only thing that makes them feel normal, or controls their otherwise uncontrolled psychiatric and physical symptoms. Many of the drugs discussed are therapeutically effective, and therefore are available through prescription use under the guidance of trained and licensed practitioners. Such medications can be life-saving, but should always be used with caution and under proper supervision.

Many drugs are illicit (illegal) and have no therapeutic benefit at all. They are abused simply to obtain the effect of that drug. Reasons vary, ranging from euphoria to seeking the sensation of religious or mystical experiences. There are far more drugs than can ever be included in these appendices. The purpose of these appendices is to address the most common drugs and drug classes, the ones we are most likely to see within the United States culture. The appendices include the most common names of drugs, the most common street names, the most common effects of the drugs, etc. Despite an attempt to be thorough, there will always be new names, new drugs, or simply information that was too much in depth to include in this book.

Finally, where applicable each appendix includes brief descriptions of safer alternatives to the drugs, or treatment options for dependence on those drugs. In general, if there is truly an addiction problem, an alternative medication will not resolve the problem of addiction, and treatment programs guided by addiction counselors and other qualified professionals are essential for addiction recovery.

The appendices are presented with the more commonly abused drugs first. Then I include an appendix with information regarding the actions of various neurotransmitters, all of which is essential to understanding addiction.

APPENDIX A

Alcohol

Alcohol has been around for millennia. The celebration of alcohol use and the tragic stories of its abuse fills our literature. Even scriptures record many episodes in which alcohol played a negative role in the lives of people. Societies (including the United States) have gone to great lengths to limit or abolish the abuse of alcohol, attempting to reduce its devastating effects upon its citizens. Temperance societies sprang up throughout history to decry the evils of the drink. Yet, few people listened to the warnings, and attempts to regulate or eliminate alcohol use are viciously resisted. Even when legislation is successful in making alcohol illegal, black markets provide ample supply to the wanting and the addicted, a testament to its potent effect upon people and its power over cultures. Early in my training, I heard an addiction specialist refer to alcohol as a "dirty drug", meaning that it triggers so many different reward centers and chemical pathways in the brain that there is no simple way to treat alcohol addiction. We cannot just block the receptor that it effects, or substitute something for it. Not only does it affect many different pathways, alcohol readily passes into the brain, and it is very toxic. Immediately upon consumption, the body breaks it down into other compounds, and the liver removes those compounds as quickly as it can. However, there is a maximum capacity at which the body can eliminate alcohol. Because of this, the amount of alcohol consumed is somewhat predictive of blood alcohol levels. In turn, blood alcohol levels have a somewhat predictive effect on the body, even though there is a great deal of variation in how one drink may affect an individual.

ALCOHOL EFFECTS
Progression – low levels to high levels

decreased inhibitions
sensation of warmth, flushing of skin
mild impairment of judgement
more social
slurring of speech
loss of problem solving ability
emotional instability
inappropriate social interactions
loss of fine motor skills
double vision
lethargy
loss of gross motor skills
staggering gait, slurred speech
memory loss
stupor
deep sleep
coma
incontinent
respiratory suppression
low blood pressure
vomiting
aspiration of vomit
breathing stops
circulation collapses

SHORT-TERM RISKS OF ALCOHOL CONSUMPTION

Motor vehicle accidents
Injuries
Burns
Violence
Suicide
Homicide
Sexual Assault
High risk behaviors, drugs, sex
Alcohol toxicity

ALCOHOL WITHDRAWAL SYMPTOMS

anxiety
tremors
high blood pressure
rapid heart rate
irritability
agitation
seizures
delirium tremens
nausea and vomiting
headache
insomnia
hallucinations
confusion
sweating
fevers

Every person metabolizes alcohol differently, thus the effects upon them vary. For example, many Asians and many women do not metabolize alcohol as well. One drink could make them quite ill. In reality, they are the fortunate ones. Some individuals boast about their capacity to "hold their beer." This has been a badge of honor in many cultures for centuries. The real truth is individuals who can tolerate a higher amount of alcohol are the most likely to become addicted to it, and develop all of the subsequent problems associated with alcoholism. For most people, delayed reaction times and other symptoms of inebriation kick in at or below a blood alcohol level of 0.08 g/dl. Highly intoxicated people have blood levels exceeding 0.12 g/dl, and those whose blood alcohol level reaches the 0.4 g/dl range or above can die. A frightening truth people don't realize, especially our youth is that what one person can drink and recover from can be lethal to another person. Also, chronic use does drive tolerance just as it does with other drugs. Over time, the body does increase in its ability to metabolize and to tolerate alcohol, but at a huge price to our system and organs. During an emergency room rotation in Detroit I had a patient who came in to have a laceration on his eyebrow stitched. As I sewed, we had a good conversation. He was completely conversant and coherent. His blood alcohol level came back at 0.64 g/dl, well past a lethal level.

Animal cells exposed to alcohol die. Alcohol is used as a cleaning agent in health care environments because it is highly toxic to living organisms. Yet we drink this? Most of the tissues in the body will regenerate if they are harmed. For example, the liver will repeatedly repair the damage done by alcohol and other toxins, but the body and its organs can be destroyed beyond the point of repair over time. When the body loses its means of removing toxins and poisons from our system, death follows.

Alcohol is also neurotoxic, meaning it kills nerve cells, which are the slowest tissue in the body to regenerate or repair. This is why our brain is so well protected. There is a solid bone casing to guard against external damage, and a tissue barrier (called the blood-brain barrier) which keeps harmful things away from the brain tissues, such as viruses, bacteria, and toxic chemicals. However, anything that can dissolve through fat (fat soluble) can pass right into the brain. This includes alcohol, marijuana, caffeine, nicotine, and many other chemicals of abuse.

All of these chemicals of abuse have shown a direct impact on neuron development in the brain. Some, such as alcohol, are simply killers. Brain cells die as a direct result of exposure to alcohol, and though the brain has a remarkable degree of plasticity (the ability to regenerate and compensate), in adults this happens by the development of new neuronal pathways, not by the regrowth of destroyed tissues. The bottom line is, alcohol destroys the brain.

Interestingly, the risks associated with alcohol use are not just from consuming it. Withdrawal from alcohol is also neurotoxic. We have learned from our studies of alcohol abuse and how to treat it, that the effects of alcohol withdrawal can be deadly. Detoxification is an extremely dangerous condition, and unlike most drugs of abuse, can be life threatening. Seizures, delirium tremens, and death are all a risk. When an individual repeatedly withdraws and relapses, each withdrawal increases in severity and presents an even greater danger to the patient. Thus, we generally detox alcoholics under close supervision, with the support of medications. Each withdrawal also tends to get worse in the severity and danger of the withdrawal. With the fourth and fifth detoxification of a chronic alcoholic, the risk of seizures dramatically increases.

Moreover, the list of chronic diseases associated with alcohol use is extensive. Perhaps more than with most drugs of abuse, alcohol impacts many people around the abuser, in terms of accidents, physical and emotional abuse, etc. Intoxication is a dangerous condition. It changes the way people think and act, and how the body functions.

Alcohol is powerfully addictive to those who are susceptible. Even if a person is not genetically prone to alcoholism, regular use of alcohol can lead to an overwhelming addiction. At one time, I knew a young woman in treatment, who after several days complained of illness to the point she had to be taken to the emergency room for an evaluation. While there, she stole two bottles of rubbing alcohol, and proceeded to drink a large part of one before she was caught. Another man began drinking the alcohol-based hand cleansers. Many people drink Nyquil in large amounts for the alcohol it contains. Others drink colognes in search of alcohol. With deadly results, some people have tried antifreeze and wood alcohol.

In small amounts, such as the accidental consumption of fermented foods or liquids, the body is capable of processing the alcohol without harming our organs or nerves, but on the whole, the human body was not meant to deal with alcohol. It is clear, based upon the damage caused by alcohol, that it is a toxin. Our bodies are not built to detoxify alcohol other than in emergent and temporary situations. The symptoms of alcohol exposure are those of chemical toxicity, and illness. Unfortunately, those symptoms—inebriation and intoxication—are the very reasons humans seek to use this drug. We all should take note that toxic is the root of intoxication.

Due to the long history of alcohol abuse, and the progress of medical care, we now have many ways to treat intoxication, detoxification, and even medications to help prevent relapses. Benzodiazepines and barbiturates have long been used to successfully prevent the life-threatening dangers of detoxification, effectively alleviating the risk of seizures and delirium tremens (DT's).

Despite medical advances, detoxification requires a safe environment such as a residential treatment program or hospitalization. The use of benzodiazepines and barbiturates in treating acute withdrawal can increase the risk of relapse if not properly administered and monitored. Both of these drugs are addictive, and may potentiate the effects of, and addictiveness of, alcohol.

Repeatedly going through alcohol withdrawals can increase the risk of seizures with each subsequent withdrawal. Research in treating alcohol withdrawal with less addictive seizure medications, like valproic acid, carbamazapine, and gabapentin is ongoing. The effectiveness of these medications in preventing complications during withdrawals and in reducing the incidence of relapse has been promising, but they still need to be given in a safe, supervised environment.

LONG-TERM RISKS OF ALCOHOL CONSUMPTION

Social instability
Family dysfunction
Depression
Anxiety
Insomnia
Liver cirrhosis
Cardiomyopathy (enlarged heart)
Heart arrhythmias
High blood pressure
Anemia
Ulcers
Pancreatitis
Strokes
Memory loss
Dementia
Liver cancer
Stomach cancer
Mouth, larynx, and throat cancers
Esophageal cancer
Colon cancer
Breast cancer
School failure
Unemployment
Addiction
Fetal Alcohol Syndrome
Seizures
Gout
Nerve damage
Incontinence
Constipation
Weakness
Numbness and burning
Sexual dysfunction
Abdominal pain
Chronic diarrhea
Sexually transmitted diseases

Common medications used in treating alcoholism

Benzodiazepines:

Benzodiazepines (commonly called "benzos") prevent seizures, thus protecting patients during the withdrawal phase of alcohol detoxification. They are also very effective at decreasing anxiety and helping insomnia. Alcoholics often drink to get themselves to sleep, and then are unable to sleep without the alcohol. During the short-term detoxification process, benzos are very helpful. As noted previously, benzos can potentiate the effects of alcohol, and are often combined in drug "cocktails" with alcohol, providing an effect more potent than either the alcohol or the benzos by themselves. This is a very dangerous combination, as they are both "downers," sedating the body and its functions. Giving any alcoholic benzos to take home is very dangerous. In skilled hands, benzos help patients safely detox from chronic alcohol use, and are currently the standard for acute alcohol withdrawal.

For a list and discussion of benzos please see Appendix E.

Barbiturates:

Barbiturates are older than benzos, but have very similar qualities relative to the detoxification of alcohol. Phenobarbital is a barbiturate often used in alcohol detox. It has anti-seizure effects, but is not quite as effective at alleviating some of the other withdrawal symptoms as the benzos. In addition, barbiturates are a little more difficult to manage and use safely. The same concerns about potentiation and relapse exist as with the benzos. With the research being done on new medications, barbiturates will likely become less and less common for alcohol detoxification.

Acamprosate:

Marketed under the name Campral, this drug effects the GABA and glutamate receptors, thus decreases the patient's cravings for alcohol and reduces the risk of a relapse. Studies clearly showed the drug curtails cravings in many patients, but not in everyone. For some, it has no effect. Another problem with this medication is very poor digestive absorption. Each tablet contains 333 milligrams of the drug and a patient must take two tablets three times per day to achieve a therapeutic level. Six tablets a day becomes fairly expensive, but for some patients the benefits are worth the cost.

Naltrexone:

Naltrexone is an opiate blocker and used in treating both opiate and alcohol addictions. As previously noted, alcohol is a "dirty drug", that affects many different receptors in the brain, including opiate receptors. Blocking the opiate receptors for some alcoholics results in a decreased craving for alcohol and becomes a tremendous help in their recovery. Again, there are some people this drug does little to help. Trial of the drug can determine if it will work for each person. Generic testing is becoming more available to assess the efficacy of medications for individual patients.

Happily, the generic form of naltrexone in a 50-mg tablet is only taken once a day, which makes it cost effective. The brand name of the tablet, ReVia, is much more expensive. There is also an injectable form called Vivitrol, which costs more, but is administered once a month and may be a better choice for certain individuals. The patient receives the benefits of consistent treatment that is not dependent on daily compliance or remembering to take the medication. As a complete opiate blocker, naltrexone is very useful in the treatment of opiate addiction, but with alcoholics, it works to reduce cravings for some individuals.

Disulfiram:

Marketed as Anatabuse, disulfiram slows down acetaldehyde dehydrogenase, the enzyme that helps us break down alcohol in our system to less toxic byproducts. Acetaldehyde is a product of many processes, including natural processes. It can be found in car emissions, breads, coffees, plant products, ripe fruits, groundwater, and is a product of the partial oxygenation of ethanol. As it can be found in so many places, it is logical that our bodies would have a means to break it down into a less harmful substance, acetic acid (the primary component of vinegar).

Consumption of alcohol, on the other hand, can easily overload this metabolic system. The partial oxidation of ethanol, leading to large amounts of acetaldehyde, may be responsible for many of the negative side effects of alcohol, including hangovers. By inhibiting that enzyme, we suffer the effects of an increasing toxicity of alcohol. This results in vomiting, headaches, dizziness, confusion, flushing of the skin, shortness of breath, visual disturbances, rapid heart rate, and more. Essentially, it makes drinking alcohol a very bad experience.

The downsides of the medication are that it does not reduce cravings for alcohol, and it has to be taken every day to work. Unfortunately, it produces such severe illness when alcohol is consumed, people simply choose to skip the medication and go drink to satisfy their cravings. So, to be effective in the treatment of alcoholism, this medication requires close monitoring. Under observed, daily administration, it becomes a strong deterrent.

Patients have to be very careful when taking this drug, though. If they use alcohol in any form—hand sanitizers, colognes, or other alcohol based substances--within the previous twelve hours, they could become ill if they take the disulfiram.

APPENDIX B

Tobacco/Nicotine

Nicotine is the chemical in tobacco products which leads to the dependence upon tobacco. Nicotine is primarily obtained by smoking tobacco products, though many people "chew" tobacco, which in essence means they suck on the tobacco, pulling the nicotine and other compounds out of the tobacco with their saliva. It is absorbed through the mucous membranes of the mouth, and in some cases swallowed with the saliva. Smoking tobacco generally takes the forms of cigarettes, pipes, or cigars, being inhaled and rapidly absorbed through the lungs into the blood.

The American Lung Association, as well as many others, identify smoking (tobacco use) as the single "...most important source of preventable morbidity (disease and illness) and premature mortality (death) worldwide." They also report an estimated 443,000 American lives lost each year, as well as an average cost of $4,260 per adult smoker in the United States per year (based on 2004 statistics). [1]

Smoking has been well studied, relative to the cost and other effects upon society. Remarkably, people continue to smoke. As with other drugs, there are many reasons people start smoking, but essentially one reason they do not quit: they are addicted. Many people will argue this, and say they can stop at any time (much like marijuana use—though it is more addicting than marijuana), yet while saying this, they are not willing to give up their source of nicotine. It seems incredibly unlikely that so many people would continue to habitually do something so well-documented to be so dangerous unless an addictive, brain-rewarding process reinforced their behavior. Certainly, social cues and habituation contribute to these issues also, but there is no question about the addictive nature of nicotine.

DISEASES LINKED TO TOBACCO

- COPD
- Emphysema
- Chronic bronchitis
- Coronary artery disease
- Stroke
- Abdominal aortic aneurysm
- Acute myeloid leukemia
- Cataracts
- Pneumonia
- Periodontitis
- Cancers of:
    - Bladder
    - Esophagus
    - Larynx
    - Lung
    - Mouth
    - Tongue
    - Throat
    - Cervix
    - Kidney
    - Stomach
    - Pancreas
- Infertility
- Peripheral vascular disease
- Peptic ulcer disease
- Blood clots

Recently, smoking in public places has come under attack. The knowledge gained over the past few decades about the damage done to non-smokers by second-hand smoke inhalation has led to laws which ultimately make it more inconvenient to smoke. Smoke-free zones are growing, and most physicians tell patients to give up smoking if there are children in the house. Of course, the most common report is, "I only smoke outside," or "I only smoke in my bedroom." Sadly, this is generally not true, and children are exposed. Studies show it really makes little difference where the smoking occurs. Children in smoking households have a higher rate of upper respiratory infections compared to children in non-smoking households.

SMOKERS DIE EARLIER [1]

13.2 years for men
14.5 years for women

The list of diseases smoking causes or contributes to is quite extensive and the statistics regarding smoking could fill quite a few books. The American Lung Association has an information-filled web site, and has done a remarkable job of summarizing the data regarding the hazards and effects of smoking. Perhaps some people reading this book will need little convincing of the dangers of smoking. However, many good people are trapped by nicotine, and do not understand why it is so difficult for them to "kick the habit." I have had many patients tell me that it was easier to stop their "hard drugs," like cocaine, or heroine, than to stop smoking. Everybody's addictive susceptibilities are different. One person may be able to quit smoking with a simple decision. For another nicotine is terribly addictive and very difficult to overcome.

To understand this powerful drug, which is one of society's costliest addictions, we need to examine how it works on the body. Nicotine is a stimulant that functions in different ways. One effect is it causes a direct release of adrenaline into the brain, making the user very "alert" or aware. Yet, oddly at the same time, it also has a calming effect on the individual. The results are dose dependent by using short puffs, deep inhalations, or by frequency of use. At low doses, nicotine can cause a release of dopamine, thus making the user relaxed. However, at increasing doses, nicotine becomes a greater stimulant by triggering releases of serotonins and endorphins. The endorphin release can be substantial enough to reduce pain. Nicotine also activates many other neurotransmitters and chemical signals in the body. In high doses, this drug can be dangerous, and even lethal.

Smoking any drug rapidly provides the desired effect, because the drug is quickly absorbed through the lungs, into the blood, and carried directly to the brain. It only takes 7-10 seconds for the nicotine to reach the brain after tobacco smoke is inhaled. This poses some difficulties when treating nicotine addiction. Nicotine replacement has been one of the mainstays of therapy, though with limited effectiveness.

Nicotine is typically replaced using gum, a lozenge, or a patch. These forms provide a much slower delivery system. As a result, the person using them feels much less benefit from the replacement. The nicotine takes longer to reach the blood and the brain, does not produce a rapid sensation of effectiveness, and because it rises slowly and then fades gradually away, it simply gives a different effect than nicotine inhaled.

Recently e-cigarettes have become common. These use a battery to heat an electric element which heats a solution containing nicotine. There is limited regulation on this right now, and there is both promise and concern. Nicotine itself is far less dangerous when delivered without the tar and contaminants in tobacco products. Therefore, this form of nicotine replacement may decrease the costs and the severity of chronic diseases associated with smoking. However, the FDA is apprehensive about what is in the solution, and intends to make sure it is safe for the consumer. Regulation may come forward regarding the use and distribution of e-cigarettes.

Individuals should be worried about e-cigarette use regardless of regulations. As I stated, nicotine is highly addictive and the easy availability of e-cigarettes can cause a surge in nicotine dependence. Especially if e-cigarettes are perceived by our youth to be another "safe" drug like marijuana. The culture of being cool if you "smoke" may see a rebirth.

Nicotine addiction, even minus the negatives of tobacco, is still dangerous to the user and destructive to the body. One addictive process can trigger or lead to other addictive processes, and the effects of nicotine addiction have far-reaching consequences. Smoking has been shown to be particularly problematic to women of child-bearing age. Certainly, everyone has heard of the risks to the unborn child if the mother is a smoker. Smoking causes damage to the placenta, decreasing the flow of healthy nutrients and oxygen to the developing fetus. Smoking mothers are more prone to deliver prematurely and to have low birth weight babies.

Smoking in conjunction with estrogen is also a very dangerous combination. There is a high risk of developing blood clots in women who are taking estrogen containing birth control or hormone replacement medications while smoking. Birth control alone slightly increases that risk, and smoking alone does also, but the combination of the two introduces a dramatic elevation of the risk of developing blood clots. Blood clots can form in many places. They can damage any organ where they may lodge. Two more well-known examples include the brain (causing a stroke) and the lungs (pulmonary embolus). Blood clot formation can be fatal.

Though there is research showing nicotine has some potential benefit in memory and performance tests on patients with Alzheimer's Disease, schizophrenia, and ADHD[2], the controlled use of a drug for therapeutic results is vastly different than the repeated use of a drug due to an addiction. Do not justify abuse by thinking it may have some positive effect.

To try and help treat nicotine addiction, recent developments in nicotine vaccines are promising. The vaccine induces the production of antibodies against nicotine. The theory being, if

EFFECTS OF NICOTINE

Spasm of the airways
Nausea
Vomiting
Fever
Dry mouth
Heartburn and reflux
Headaches
Lightheadedness
Sleep abnormalities
Irritability
Increased blood pressure
Increased heart rate
Irregular heart rate
Tightness in chest
Runny nose
Artery constriction in heart
Insulin resistance
Throat irritation
Anxiety
Muscle pain
Confusion
Seizures
Exhaustion
Tissue damage to airways

NICOTINE REPLACEMENT PRODUCTS

nicotine inhaled	e-cigarettes
	Nicotrol Inhaler
nicotine nasal	Nicotrol NS
nicotine transdermal	Nicoderm CQ
nicotine transmucosal	Nicorette Gum
	Nicorette Lozenge
	Nicorette Mini Lozenge

SMOKING CESSATION PRODUCTS

bupropion hydrochloride	Budeprion SR
	Buproban
	Wellbutrin SR
	Zyban
varenicline	Chantix

NICOTINE WITHDRAWAL [3]

Headache	Insomnia
Nausea	Irritability
Constipation	Difficult concentrating
Diarrhea	Anxiety
Slow heart rate	Depression
Low blood pressure	Increased hunger
Fatigue	Desire for sweets
Drowsiness	Tobacco cravings

someone smokes, the antibodies will attack and immobilize the nicotine before it can pass from the blood into the brain. So far, the vaccines do not produce high enough antibody levels to block nicotine effects well, though trials have shown vaccines do enhance smoking cessation rates. Newer methods are being studied in hopes of introducing higher levels of nicotine antibodies.

Medications have also been developed to try and combat cravings and the desire for nicotine by adjusting the reward neurotransmitters within the brain. Bupropion (branded Budeprion, Buproban, Forfivo, Wellbutrin, Zyban) decreases cravings for nicotine, and was marketed for smoking cessation. In some cases, it did effectively decrease nicotine cravings, but was not as successful as had been hoped. Varenicline, marketed as Chantix, has been more successful in the treatment of nicotine addiction, despite the reported side effects in some people — rare, worsening of depression, and vivid bizarre dreams. Treatment using Chantix started with introducing the drug at an escalating dose for one week, and then stopping the smoking completely. Variations of this have followed, but overall if a person can take it without the side effects noted above, it seems to be very effective. Again, however, the person using it must simply have a solid determination to stop smoking, as neither bupropion or varenicline will simply make someone stop smoking. Having said that, I have had two cases where the individual taking the medicines became ill every time they smoked, so in that sense, the medicines did make them stop smoking.

As with all addictions, in addition to the withdrawal symptoms caused by the nicotine dependence, there are social and habitual triggers. Where a person smokes, what they do while they smoke, what they eat when they smoke, who they are with when they smoke, and where they take a break at work for smoking all are examples of cues that trigger a desire to smoke. These all must be accounted for when attempting to quit smoking. Coffee in the morning while smoking and reading the newspaper is a common trigger. Smoking while driving is another. As soon as the person gets in the car, smells the cigarettes, and puts one hand on the wheel, they will begin to crave that cigarette. Such social cues must be considered, and will persist long beyond the last withdrawals from the actual nicotine.

Acupuncture, massage, hypnosis, and other methods of changing the body's response to the nicotine and to the triggers have shown promise in reducing the risks of relapse to smoking. A combination of both medication, counseling, and "alternative" treatments such as these could be very promising for both cessation and long-term abstinence.

APPENDIX C

Cannabinoids

Marijuana is the most well-know of the cannabinoids. It is the most widely-used illicit drug in the world. Marijuana use increased steadily among teens in the early nineties, then dropped in the early 2000's, but then resurged in 2008.[1] Despite the perception of marijuana risk and harm being at an all-time low, there is more and more evidence that the use of marijuana does change brain structure and function in adolescents. The average age of first use has also declined (meaning kids are using it earlier and earlier).

MARIJUANA (MARIHUANA)

Also known as:
Cannabis (Cannabinoids)

Most psychoactive component:
Tetrahydrocannabinol (THC)

Contains at least 480 other compounds in the marijuana plant.

Marijuana is now more in the public eye than it has been in decades because of the ongoing debate regarding the legalization of its use. The extent of those debates is far beyond the capacity of this book. However, several issues can be boiled down to simple concepts, to understand the impact of marijuana.

Proponents of marijuana legalization state it has no ill effects, and it does not lead to the use of other drugs. Yet, a review of medical literature supports the concept of marijuana as a "gateway"

Percent of Students Reporting Use of Marijuana in Past Year, by Grade [1]

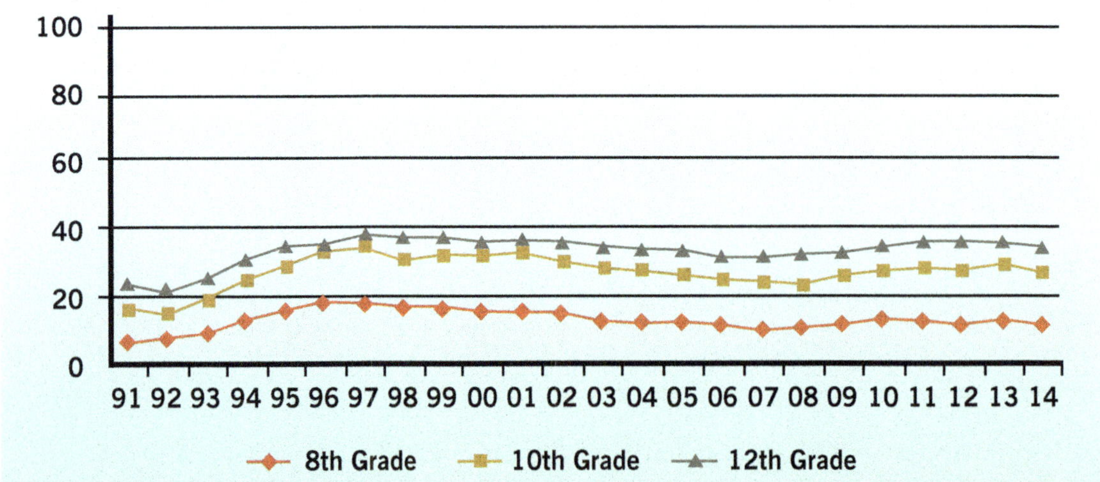

drug. The debate about what a "gateway drug" really means, and whether or not marijuana truly is a gateway drug, seems endless. What can be said is that marijuana is being consistently used at a younger age than other drugs, and people who use multiple drugs tend to use marijuana as one of those drugs. So, arguing whether one leads to the other, or whether other factors contribute to the use of marijuana is pointless. The fact remains, that use of marijuana frequently leads to the use of other drugs. This may be due to the desire to find a "higher" high, or possibly because it is a part of the culture of drug use, with increased availability of other drugs. There could be many other reasons why marijuana is used early. Simply put, marijuana is part of the drug culture. Where marijuana is used, other drugs are very often used. When other drugs are used, marijuana is very often found in the mix.

There is also a certain decision process that persists amongst us as humans, and once one risky behavior has been tried, we find it much easier to try another. This is certainly true with drug use. Marijuana also decreases some of our natural inhibitions, and like other drugs leads to more risk taking.

Marijuana has also been blamed for a much-debated condition called an "a-motivational syndrome." This simply means the user becomes so relaxed about life in general, they quit worrying about other things which are important, such as school, work, and family. Many people dispute this, but so many times an addict in recovery has explained to me how their marijuana use led to them dropping out of school, losing their job, and just not caring about any of it.

STREET NAMES [2]

Marijuana
Mary Jane
MJ
Reefer
Pot
Weed
Grass
Dope
Ganja
Hash
Herb
Aunt Mary
Skunk
Boom
Chronic
Cheeba
Blunt
Ashes
Atshitshi
Baby Bhang
Bammy
Blanket
Bo-Bo
Bobo Bush
Bomber
Boom
Broccoli
Cripple
Dagga
Dinkie Dow
Ding
Dona Juana (or Juanita)
Flower, Flower Tops
Ganja
Gasper
Giggle Smoke
Good Giggles
Good Butt
Hot Stick
Jay
Jolly Green
Joy Smoke,
Joy Stick
Roach

Many people say to me marijuana is misunderstood and harmless. They claim that other than being born after marijuana became illegal, they've done nothing wrong in their recreational use of the drug. Marijuana had no ill effect on them.

When I ask about their experiences during this drug use, I find their stories enlightening. Even while denying any ill effects from marijuana, they tell me of hallucinations, such as thinking the government has bugged the shed where they smoke. Some said they heard voices while under the influence, and others participate in stupid, sometimes very dangerous activities because they thought God told them to do so. Some experienced moments of extreme empathy, and acting upon those feelings caused major social problems. Some heard songs that weren't on their audio devices. Harmless?

When we look at the long-term studied effects of marijuana, we learn of the problems with marijuana use. True, it is safer than most drugs because it is almost impossible to die from overdose or from dangerous withdrawal symptoms. However, recently, with the legalization of marijuana resulting in escalating marijuana use, we are seeing a condition called cannabinoid hyperemesis syndrome, with sudden severe episodes of nausea and vomiting, in contrast to the typical anti-nausea effect of marijuana. Additionally, the incidence of developing psychiatric problems (particularly schizophrenia) is higher with chronic marijuana use than it is for non-users. We also know the lifetime rate of developing dependence on marijuana is 9%. Thus, anyone that uses marijuana has a 9% chance of becoming dependent on it, and end up being at risk for the long-term effects of using marijuana. Studies comparing marijuana and tobacco smoke have also shown comparable risks relative to lung damage and long-term respiratory problems, though those effects seem to be with higher doses of marijuana use.

Additionally, there is very clear research showing loss of executive functions of the brain the longer one uses marijuana. That functional loss is even more dramatic when the use of marijuana starts at a younger age. Those who smoke marijuana have a drop in their IQ compared to those who have never smoked. Any drug use, including marijuana, has been shown to damage the ability to make decisions regarding appropriate and inappropriate behaviors. Impulsivity also increases.

I must add there is a legitimate medical use for cannabinoids. They do help decrease nausea and vomiting (when used in controlled doses), and stimulate appetite. Several disease conditions cause a loss of appetite, and in those conditions the patient may get weaker and weaker, or be unable to obtain the protein they need to heal. Dronabinol (marketed as Marinol) is a cannabinoid that has been formulated into a pill form. It currently has an FDA indication for nausea and vomiting related to chemotherapy in cancer patients, and for loss of appetite and weight loss in AIDS-related complications.

Marijuana has been shown to decrease pressure within the eye, potentially being a treatment for glaucoma. It also has some pain-relieving characteristics. Additionally, it may increase some parameters in lung function, though probably temporarily. Many people also use it for anxiety relief. Unfortunately, many of the people who use it for anxiety relief

EFFECTS OF CANNABINOIDS

- Dry Mouth
- Sensation of cold
- Red eyes
- Decreased pressure in eyes
- Relaxation of muscles
- Increased heart rate
- Increased appetite
- Decrease blood pressure
- Impaired short-term memory
- Hallucinations

LONG TERM EFFECTS

- Increased risk of psychiatric illness
- Decreased IQ when used as adolescent
- Inhibition of neuralgic development in adolescents
- Addictive potential

SLANG TERMS FOR MARIJUANA USE AND ABUSE [4]

Blast (blast a roach, blast a stick, blast a joint) * Blow one's roof * Blowing smoke * Blow a stick * Boot the gong * Airhead (marijuana user) * Bite one's lips * Bogart * Hi the Hay * Burn one * Fire it up * Get a gage up * Get the wind * Fly Mexican Airlines * Mow the grass * Tea party * Toke * Torch up have the anxiety because of long-term marijuana or other drug use. Sadly, like so many other drugs, prolonged use followed by the absence of the drug leads to acute and chronic anxiety syndromes. However, there are other medicines effective in performing these same therapeutic effects, so it makes no sense to use marijuana when it can lead to so many other problems.

In my assessment, despite potential medical uses, the risks of legalizing marijuana under the current circumstances is too great. There are far too many deleterious effects at this point. The American Society of Addiction Medicine has taken a clear stand against the legalization of marijuana until further research is done. Many others involved in the research of marijuana and its effects have taken similar stands, primarily because of the addictive potential and the damage to the developing brain in individuals younger than their mid-twenties.

WITHDRAWAL SYMPTOMS [5]

Anxiety
Mood swings
Cravings
Depression
Insomnia
Nightmares
Vivid dreams
"using" dreams
Change in appetite
Weight loss or gain
Headaches
Loss of sense of humor
Loss of sex drive
Shakiness
Dizziness

MARIJUANA LACED WITH SOME SORT OF NARCOTIC [3]

Amp Joint, Dust, Dusting *

MARIJUANA AND HEROIN:

Atom Bomb, A-Bomb, Canade, Woola, Woolie, Woo-Woo, Brown *

MARIJUANA AND PCP:

Ace, Bohd, Chips, Frios, Zoom *

MARIJUANA AND LSD:

Beast, LBJ *

MARIJUANA AND CRACK:

Buda, Butter, Crack Back, Fry Daddy, Geek, Juice Joint *

MARIJUANA AND COCAINE:

Banano, Basuco, Bush, Chase, Cocktail, Cocoa Puff, Hooter, Jim Jones, Lace *

MARIJUANA AND ALCOHOL:

Herb and Al

EFFECTS ON LIFE

Research clearly demonstrates that marijuana has the potential to cause problems in daily life or make a person's existing problems worse. In fact, heavy marijuana users generally report lower life satisfaction, poorer mental and physical health, relationship problems, and less academic and career success compared to their peers who came from similar backgrounds. For example, marijuana use is associated with a higher likelihood of dropping out from school. Several studies also associate workers' marijuana smoking with increased absences, tardiness, accidents, workers' compensation claims, and job turnover. [6]

APPENDIX D

Opiates and Opioids

COMMON OPIATES/OPIOIDS IN THE U.S.

Generic	Brand
codeine	Many formulations
fentanyl	Abstral
	Fentora
	Actin
	Lazanda
	Onsolis
	Duragesic
	Sublimaze
	Subsys
hydromorphone	Dilaudid,
	Dilaudid-HP
	Exalgo
levorphanol	Levo-Dromoran
meperidine	Demerol
methadone	Dolphin
	Methadose
morphine sulfate	Avinza
	Kadian
	MS Contin
	Oramorph SR
	Roxanne
nalbuphine	Nubain

Opium has been around for thousands of years. The word opium derives from the Greek word opion, but the use of opium far predates the Greeks. Opium is extracted from the Opium poppy, or Papaver Somniferum, by either slicing the seed pod and collecting the sap that drains, or extracting it from the dried plant. The terms opiate and opioid are somewhat confusing, and often interchanged. Morphine is the primary product of the poppy. Many other opiates are derived from the poppy. Opiate, then, is the term used for the products derived completely or partially from the poppy or from morphine. Opioid is the term used for synthetically manufactured drugs that also work on the opiate receptors in the body. There are several different receptors in the body which respond to opiates and opioids. The action of the particular drug and which receptor(s) it acts upon determines the specific characteristics of the drug.

For the sake of simplicity, I will refer to all opiates and opioids simply as opiates. It is not really necessary to refer to the classes separately, as they are all potentially addictive, and have similar characteristics. I will list the different drugs under their class, but otherwise our discussion of addiction does not need to differentiate between those medications derived from opium and synthetic opioids. Narcotic is yet another term used to describe the opiate-derived pain medications.

Opiates are an effective and beneficial class of medications. They are primarily used for pain relief. They change the way the brain perceives pain, lessening the intensity of pain, and increasing a person's tolerance of pain. However, they also produce sedation and decrease respiratory drive, which results in the risk of "overdose" if too much is taken. Opiate overdose simply causes a cessation of breathing. Another significant side effect is constipation, which can become a severe problem. Cough suppression is yet another effect of opiates, and is used in several common cough syrups.

Unfortunately, euphoria is also a side effect of opiates. The sense of well-being produced by a large dose of opiates, particularly in an opiate naive person, is one of the biggest draws for opiate abuse. The euphoria and sedation combined cause such a sense of well-being that the misuse of the drug often leads to addiction.

Opiates are the most effective means of acute pain control we currently know, at least medicinally. They are tremendously effective. If used in appropriate situations (meaning for people who are truly in pain), they rarely lead to an escalation of dose and addiction, though if used for prolonged periods they almost always lead to a dependence, which leads in turn to withdrawals if stopped.

Appropriate use of narcotics is difficult to judge. Many practitioners are not trained well regarding the risks of narcotic use. Even if they are trained well, it is incredibly hard to truly assess another person's levels of pain. Often patients come in to the office complaining of severe pain, and pleading for relief. Pain is a terrible thing to live with. Pain is also a very subjective issue. A practitioner is dependent on a patient's report of pain, as it is difficult to test for pain, or to quantify pain or pain tolerance within the setting of an office visit. Pain is also experienced very differently by each individual. Some people suffer tremendous pain with very small injuries, whereas others do not perceive much pain from very serious injuries. For example, I knew one man who completely crushed the end half of his finger in a log splitter, shattering the bones, and ripping off part of the finger. He took one or two low dose hydrocodone for a couple of days and had adequate pain control. I have known other people who have demanded high dose narcotics after receiving a simple laceration in an area with less sensitivity than the hand.

Despite the variation in people's perception of pain, there is a growing need for pain control. In our society, as we live longer and longer, we see the development of more chronic pain syndromes. With age comes more severe arthritis and other degenerative processes that result in pain. We also

COMMON OPIATES/OPIOIDS IN THE U.S. *(continued)*

Generic	Brand
oxycodone	OxyContin
	OxyFast
	Roxicodone
	Oxecta
oxymorphone	Opana
	Opana ER
pentazocine	Talwin
propoxyphene	Darvon, Darvon-N
tapentadol	Nucynta. Nucynta ER
	Nucynta ER
tramadol	Rybix ODT
	Ryzolt
	Ultram
	Ultram ER
	ConZip
butorphanol	Stadol NS
	Nubain
	Stadol
buprenorphine	Butrans
	Buprenex

"In 2007, the U.S. Substance Abuse and Mental Health Services reported that 21% of people over 12 years of age used prescription painkillers non-medically." [1]

COMMON OPIATE COMBINATION DRUGS IN THE U.S.

Generic	Brand
morphine sulfate/naltrexone	
pentazocine/naloxone	
codeine/guaifenesin	
codeine/acetaminophen	Tylenol #3
	Tylenol #4
butalbital/acetaminophen/caffeine/codeine	Fioricet with codeine
butalbital/aspirin/caffeine/codeine	Fiorinol with codeine
carisoprodol/aspirin/codeine	
promethazine/codeine	Phenergan/codeine
Soma with codeine	
Tylenol with Codeine	
hydrocodone/ibuprofen	Ibudone
	Reprexain
hydrocodone/acetaminophen	Hycet
	Lorcet, Lorcet Plus
	Loretta
	Maxidone
	Norco
	Vicodin, VicodinES,
	Vicodin HP
	Zamicet
	Zodone
oxycodone/acetaminophen	Endocet
	Percocet
	Primalev
	Roxicet
	Tylox
	Xolox
	Magnacet

see the development of more cancers. Treating the pain of cancer is where narcotics have proven to be invaluable. There is little else that will adequately control the pain of cancers growing within the bones or other organs of our bodies.

In the setting of controlling end-of-life pain caused by cancer no one should ever be concerned about addiction. There are several reasons for this. First, the pain is very real and very severe, and therefore the true effect of opiate use is for pain relief and not for euphoria. The chance of addiction in this setting is very minimal. Second, if someone is dying of a cancer, and the pain is severe, no one should worry about addiction, as there is no time left to develop an addiction, particularly with true pain. What time is left should be spent as comfortably as possible,

COMMON OPIATE COMBINATION DRUGS IN THE U.S. *(continued)*

Generic	Brand
oxycodone/aspirin	Percodan
oxycodone/ibuprofen	Combunox
Propoxyphene/acetaminophen	Balacet 325
	Darvocet
tramadol/acetaminophen	Altercate
acetaminophen/caffeine/dihydrocodeine	Panlor DC
	Panlor SS
	Trezix
dihydrocodeine/aspirin/caffeine	Synagogs-DC
pentazosin/acetaminophen	Talacen

and there are plenty of medications to assure this, including both opiates and benzodiazepines. Third, there is really no other way to adequately control the pain that comes with the progression of cancer.

Because of the increasing need for opiate pain medications, the supply and access has greatly increased. Unfortunately, this production and availability of opiates led to a dramatic increase in abuse. Practitioners are ever more bombarded with patients who present with some sort of pain syndrome. It is easy to prescribe an opiate, yet few practitioners have been well-taught regarding addiction. Many readily hand out pain medicines to keep patients happy, or to avoid the inevitable confrontations with troublesome addicts. Others refuse to provide any opiates. To make it more complex, lawsuits have been filed against doctors who do not adequately control pain for patients who appear to suffer from many forms of chronic pain. For a time pain was even called "the fifth vital sign," and government entities penalized hospitals and physicians for not adequately controlling patients' pain. These factors culminated in an incredible upsurge in prescribing opiates over the first decade of this century. Now opiate abuse is epidemic. The rebound pendulum is swinging, but a little late to prevent a lot of sorrow. Yet this may lead to other problems. As the government increases regulations on opiate use, more and more physicians are afraid to prescribe pain medicines to their patients. Unfortunately, more and more patients who once received large doses of pain pills are now turning back to the cheap and readily accessible heroin, or other illicit drugs.

Differentiating a patient in true pain from a patient who has earned a personal degree in acting is difficult. Opiate addicts not only become expert actors, but when they go through opiate withdrawal they truly do experience severe pain, as well as other opiate withdrawal symptoms. Sometimes it is hard to tell between opiate withdrawal and true pain. Some of the practitioners

COMMON STREET NAMES FOR OPIATES [3]

Opium

Big O, Black Stuff, Block, Gum, Hop, Dover's Powder

Heroin

Dope, Smack, H, Train, Thunder, Black Tar, China Whitehorse, Junk, Antifreeze, Brown Sugar, Henry, Horse, Skag, Hero, Hell Dust

Fentanyl

Apache, China Girl, China White, Dance Fever, Friend, Goodfella, King Ivory, Murder 8, TNT, Tango, Cash

Morphine

M, Miss Emma, Monkey, White Stuff, Dreamer

Codeine

Schoolboy, Cough Syrup, T-three's

Hydrocodone

Vikes, Viko, Norco, Hydro

Oxycodone

Ox, Oxicotten, oxycet

COMMONLY ABUSED OPIATES [2]

codeine
morphine
methadone
fentanyl
oxycodone
oxycontin
hydrocodone
hydromorphone
hydrocodone
oxymorphone
meperidine
propoxyphene
heroin

who prescribe opiates have learned the danger signals. Signs of abuse include visiting several different doctors to get the pain medicines (doctor shopping), frequent emergency room visits, and repeat injuries (even self-inflicted). Also, those abusing the medications run out too quickly, often reporting the medications lost, or stolen. These patients tend to become very theatrical if they are not given more pain medications. They go through various stages of behaviors, from penitent, to crying and pleading, to hysterical, scared, and then to anger, and can become very threatening.

However, some people who are in true pain do lose their medications. When they suddenly find themselves with no hope of relief from their pain, they may exhibit many of the same behaviors. There are a few ways to figure out if someone is legitimately using their pain medications as prescribed, or simply abusing their prescriptions.

Most states have a board of pharmacy reporting system which will show all the controlled substances used by a patient, when they filled the prescription, and which practitioner prescribed them. Some patients jump state lines to try and fool the system. However, pharmacy reports can be accessed in different states if the practitioner wishes to do so. I have found many people getting addictive substances in surrounding states, in addition to their home state. The downside is these programs obviously do not track or account for patients who sell or buy their medications on the street.

Exploring further the effects of opiates, there is growing evidence that long-term opiate use may actually worsen chronic pain syndromes. The mechanism for this is fascinating, and most simply explained as follows: the human body produces its own opiates. These are most commonly known as endorphins and enkephalins. When we introduce a non-human opiate into our system, our body reacts by trying to produce a stable system. Our body's feedback system knows too much opiate can be detrimental to our health, to our capacity to perceive and react to pain, to our level of conscious awareness, to our capacity to breath, etc. Because of this, the body decreases the number of opiate receptors in our nerve synapses, and it reduces the amount of opiates which we make ourselves (endogenous opiates—endorphins, enkephalins, etc.).

This is the reason we see tolerance develop to opiates and other addictive drugs. The body simply reduces its own capacity to use and produce those substances, and depletes its own supply. This is also called neuroadaptation—meaning our own nervous system adapts to external abnormalities, in an attempt to maintain balance and normal function (a condition called homeostasis). Ultimately, this results in painful events causing a greater sensation of pain than they would have done if our body's natural system was working normally—a condition called hyperalgesia, or "super-pain."

Over years of opiate use, chronic pain syndromes may actually increase, despite taking the medications to relieve the pain. This is the primary reason people have a difficult time stopping opiates after they have been on them for an extended period of time. When they try to stop them, they experience severe pain, more severe than what they started with, even if the source or cause of the pain has been resolved. Aside from the hyperalgesia produced by chronic use of opiates, another reason people have so much difficulty getting off opiates is the severity of the withdrawal symptoms. Withdrawals from opiates can be terrible.

Neuroadaptation and hyperalgesia are normal processes. However, these are not necessarily the primary factors in addiction. Remember, addiction is a maladaptive behavior in which a substance is abused for the sake of a physical reward, despite the loss of critically important things in the person's life. It is very important to understand how that differs from dependence and tolerance.

The reason this is so important is that addictive behavior is very destructive. Certainly, people who have developed a tolerance, or a dependence to opiates can become addicted, and begin to participate in addictive behaviors. However, the tolerant or dependent person, if they are using the medicine as prescribed, and not resorting to criminal behavior to get more, need to understand there are ways to get off the medicine safely, and perhaps even find they do not have pain as they once thought they did. Many chronic pain syndromes will ease if an individual can stay off the narcotics for an adequate period of time. That period of time, however, is hard to predict. It might be several months, or it might be several years.

Here, it is worth noting that buprenorphine is not a typical opiate. It is listed as an opiate, but has some different and notable characteristics from the other opiates. It is used for both addiction treatment and for chronic pain.

Generally speaking, there are three reasons people maintain an addiction. First, they are using the drug to get high, or for other recreational purposes. The second reason, and the reason we usually see when they finally seek help, is to avoid the withdrawals, because eventually the recreational effects will be gone and they will find they have to constantly use in order to avoid the withdrawal. Third, some people do actually realize they are

OPIATE EFFECTS

Pain relief
Euphoria
Cough suppression
Dysphoria
Respiratory depression/arrest
Hypotension, shock
Constipation
Dependency/abuse
Nausea and vomiting
Somnolence
Dizziness
Itching
Rash
Confusion
Hallucinations
Headache
Insomnia
Hypothermia
Fevers
Urinary retention
Dry mouth (dental damage)
Sweating
Anxiety
Abdominal pain
Muscle rigidity
Paralytic ileus
Seizures
Biliary spasm
Withdrawal symptoms
Neonatal withdrawal syndrome (with use during pregnancy)
Decreased testosterone levels

OPIATE WITHDRAWAL SYMPTOMS [4]

Early symptoms of withdrawal include

Agitation
Anxiety
Muscle aches
Increased tearing
Insomnia
Runny nose
Sweating
Yawning

Late symptoms of withdrawal include

Abdominal cramping
Diarrhea
Dilated pupils
Goose bumps
Nausea
Vomiting

Opioid withdrawal reactions are very uncomfortable but are usually not life threatening.

in trouble, and are sick of living every moment enslaved to a drug, and thus they are driven to find help.

I meet many people who fall into the third category. Often, they are people who are taking opiates for pain control, and realize they are too dependent on the pain medicines, and choose to free themselves of the opiate dependence. They have become tolerant to the effects of the medicine. Their pain is as bad or worse as when they started the medication. They are taking a high dose without benefit. They cannot stop the medication on their own because of the severity of the withdrawal symptoms.

Opiate withdrawal is a terrible experience. Those who have never experienced it really cannot understand what it is like. The withdrawal results in severe pain, along with other debilitating symptoms that literally make them feel as if they will die. It is not lethal to withdraw from opiates, except in rare cases with other complicating health factors. For example, opiate withdrawal can be fatal for the fetus of a pregnant woman, or in patients with severe health problems. However, for most people who withdraw from opiates, there is no real physical danger.

Tapering down off opiates is extremely difficult, at best. Simply by the nature of an opiate, and the hyperalgesia and tolerance produced, dropping down on a dose of almost any opiate results in some withdrawal symptoms, and an increase in pain. The withdrawal is certainly less than it would be if the medicine were abruptly and completely stopped, yet more prolonged. Withdrawals can be more tolerable in small increments, but the fact that they repeat or worsen with each step becomes a significant mental and emotional battle. To confound this, there is growing evidence that the more an individual withdraws, then relapses, then withdraws, then relapses, the withdrawals may feel worse to them with each successive withdrawal if those withdrawals have been severe. Thus, individuals who have tried to quit seem to have more severe symptoms each time, and they develop a very real fear of the increasing intensity of the pain and suffering of withdrawal, being at least subconsciously aware it will likely be worse this time than it was last time. This becomes a very problematic element in helping someone come off opiates, as their fear of the withdrawal becomes incredibly powerful after multiple attempts to quit.

I have known only a handful of individuals who have taken opiates for pain long-term and have successfully tapered themselves down and off the medicines. Even more rare is the individual who uses opiates due to an addiction who has successfully tapered themselves off the opiates. Many have simply run out, or their source has dried up, and they have withdrawn completely without help, but this was not by their own choice.

Instead, addictive use tends to lead to higher and higher doses of the drug, due to the tolerance of the body, trying to reach homeostasis. Thus, the typical pattern is one of using more potent opiates over time. In light of this, it should be recognized that heroin has made a tragically successful comeback. This occurs primarily for two reasons. Other opiates no longer provide the euphoria desired, whereas heroin's delivery systems (especially injecting) gives an incredibly rapid supply of potent drug to the brain, achieving the fastest way to the greatest euphoric state. These two qualities are the primary factors sought after in drug abuse. Tragically, such a rapid and powerful delivery system also comes with a high potential for overdose and death.

The comeback of heroin due to overuse of other opiates during the first part of the twenty-first century will likely surge higher. As the supply of relatively inexpensive and easily accessible pain pills is attacked and cut back, those addicted to opiates will turn to the readily, ever present, and cheap supply of heroin. But for now, opiates are still available in abundance on the streets. Passing pills in high school hallways is common place. Substituting and mixing pills with other drugs is the purpose of "pharming parties" where everyone who comes brings bottles of any pills they can find. The drugs are dumped into a bowl, and then partiers take turns consuming various amounts of the random pills—pharmaceutical Russian roulette.

Science has shown that there is far more potential for addiction if an individual first uses at a young age. We know, for example, the younger a person starts to use tobacco, the harder it is for them to quit. This appears to be true for any addictive substance, especially used recreationally. We also know that addictive substances used before the brain has fully developed can damage the development of the brain. Adolescent brains are in the midst of pre-frontal cortex development. This happens to be the part of the brain where the concept of behavior and consequence is learned. In other words, teenagers using drugs of any sort (including marijuana) do not learn certain behaviors lead to certain consequences. The result is, when someone begins using a drug at the age of fourteen, and doesn't quit until they are thirty-four, in some ways they still behave as a fourteen-year-old, particularly in judgment of the outcomes of their behaviors and decisions.

This is true of opiates. Thus, our high school students who are passing pain pills around the hallways are stopping their brains from developing in critical ways. They will rapidly develop a tolerance to the opiates. They will shift from hydrocodone, to hydromorphone, to fentanyl, and then to heroin in search of that euphoric high they so desperately need. First, they'll take the drugs by mouth, but the tolerance leads to crushing, then snorting, then intravenous (IV) use—drawing the drug into a syringe, and injecting the drug into a vein with a small-bore needle.

IV drug use then exposes the individual to other tremendously serious hazards, overdose being only one. IV drug users are at risk for transmission of blood-borne diseases such as hepatitis, Human Immuno-Deficiency Virus (HIV) and Acquired Immune Deficiency Syndrome (AIDS). IV drug use often results in bacterial infections, which can lead to abscesses and cellulitis. Many of these infections become multi-drug resistant, such as MRSA (Methicillin Resistant

Staphylococcus Aureas). There are fewer and fewer successful treatments for this, making death a real possibility.

Intravenous needle induced blood infections can also lead to bacterial colonization and growth in various places in the body. Such an infection on a heart valve (a common place for the infection to colonize), can completely destroy the valve, then the heart, leading to death unless it is discovered and the valve is replaced before it is too late. Sepsis is another common condition, which simply means the bacteria have entered the blood stream and have begun to reproduce faster than the body's immune system can fight them. Sepsis can be rapidly fatal, leading to septic shock and death within a matter of hours if not detected and treated. Even if sepsis is caught early enough to save the victim's life, it may lead to kidney failure and the need for dialysis, or other organ failure. Virus and bacteria introduced into the blood stream can penetrate through the protective barriers surrounding the brain, leading to meningitis or encephalitis, both of which can leave an individual with brain damage, or kill them.

Within the past three to four years we have seen a new phenomenon in the world of opiate abuse. Fentanyl is a very potent pain reliever, and has been used intermittently, until 4 years ago. With the cut-back of prescription narcotic availability we not only saw a rise again in heroin and cocaine, but we started seeing more fentanyl use. Fentanyl and some super-potent chemical analogues suddenly became available from other countries. It is being ordered, shipped in to the United States, and dealers are lacing many other drugs with it. Almost any illicit drug now is at risk of being laced with fentanyl. This makes the drug much more potent, and much more dangerous. Around 2015 fentanyl deaths shot past all other opiate overdose deaths, including heroin.

Not long ago I admitted a woman to treatment who admitted she had been lacing drugs with fentanyl and selling them. She would lace every third product, whatever it was. She reports the risk of overdose was very high, but this practice made people seek her out to get drugs. Their reasoning was that if someone overdosed on her stuff then she had the good stuff, and they wanted the good stuff. Unfortunately this does not just apply to opiates, but potentially to any other drug that is sold on the street, even marijuana.

Alternatives in Pain Treatment

There are a number of alternatives for treating pain. Few are as rapidly effective or as potent as opiates, so they are much less popular, being viewed as ineffective in comparison. However, these medications, as well as other treatments can be very effective in providing pain relief. The focus of this book is not to list all the alternatives available. Yet, in warning about the risks of drug addiction, it is important to show there are alternatives. Otherwise, those suffering from pain, anxiety, and other chronic problems may give up in despair. There is ever more research which supports the effectiveness of these alternatives. Each of the topics below could fill a book, and are certainly worth researching if one desires to find methods of pain management other than opiates.

Here are some of the modalities that have good evidence for helping with chronic pain syndromes, though certainly there are others.

- Acupuncture
- Massage Therapy
- Physical Therapy (Multiple Modalities)
- Aquatic Therapy
- Biofeedback
- Hypnosis and Self-hypnosis
- Medical Nutrition Therapy

Medications:

Below is a brief review of some of the many medications that can help with pain relief. These medications have a different mechanism of effect than opiates, therefore, the way we perceive their effect is quite different. Those who have used opiates or other analgesics such as acetaminophen or ibuprofen expect to have relief of their pain within 30-60 minutes. This may not be the case with other medicines, and therefore many patients abandon these medications as ineffective.

Some of these medications alter the way the pain signals are transmitted through the nerves, while others affect the neurotransmitters between the nerves. These are different neurotransmitters that do not work on the opiate receptors. The interesting difference, however, seems to be that these medications tend to be much more effective for long-term pain management in neurogenic pain (pain caused by nerve damage). Opiates are much less effective for neurogenic pain. Still, many people want opiates—most likely because of the euphoria and sense of well-being caused by the opiate and not because of the pain relief. I have had patients say, "I still hurt, but it just makes it so I don't care about the pain."

Neurogenic pain comes in many forms. Some of the most common are spinal injuries, or disk or spine disease that pinches on a nerve. A "bad disc" with pain shooting down the leg is a good example of neurogenic pain. Limb injuries can result in chronic pain from nerve inflammation, or phantom limb pains. These conditions often respond well to the non-opiate pain medications. Nerve injuries caused by shingles, or trigeminal neuralgia, or other nerve injuries caused by inflammation such as neuropathy or neuritis, all respond well to the medications discussed below.

SNRIs (Serotonin Norepinephrine Re-uptake Inhibitors)

SNRI's are a newer class of antidepressants developed in such a way that the antidepressant effects are strong but with less of the undesirable side effects of older antidepressants. These drugs have been studied and shown to be effective for other conditions besides depression. Patients with generalized anxiety disorder, fibromyalgia, neurologic pain, and musculoskeletal pain have found relief with SNRI's, and as with other antidepressants, these are not addictive. If they are initiated in large doses, or abruptly stopped from a large dose, then they may cause symptoms of illness.

SNRI's

Generic	Brand
duloxetine	Cymbalta
venlafaxine	Effexor EffexorXR
desvenlafaxine	Pristiq

The downside to newer drugs is they are more expensive, and thus less commonly used due to expense.

TRICYCLICS

Generic	Brand
amitriptyline	Elavil
amoxapine	
clomipramine	Anafranil
desipramine	Norpramine
doxepin	Silenor
imipramine	Tofranil
	Tofranil-PM
nortryptyline	Pamela
protriptyline	Vivacity
trimipramine	Surmontil

Tricyclic Antidepressants

These are an older class of anti-depressants rarely used anymore, due to the potential side effects and reported severe drug-to-drug interactions with newer medications. These medications inhibit norepinephrine and serotonin reuptake, much like the SSRIs and SNRIs. Despite falling out of favor for depression, some are still successfully used for anxiety, and two of them are effective and safely used for chronic pain syndromes. Imipramine and amitriptyline have been used with good effect, and generally rare side effects.

Gabapentin

Gabapentin (trade name Neurontin) is an effective and commonly used pain modulator. It works by blocking proteins which allow the passage of calcium ions across the nerve membrane. In turn, this changes the release of excitatory neurotransmitters. Thus, less excitation of the post-synaptic neuron means less pain signal conduction.

Because of the decrease in excitatory signals, gabapentin can be used for some seizure conditions. However, it is very effective for any sort of neuropathic pain and widely used for pain associated with nerve inflammation or damage. For example, gabapentin is prescribed for shingles, and many who suffer pain in their hands and feet from diabetic peripheral neuropathy (nerve damage caused by diabetes) find great relief. The dosage for gabapentin is from 100 milligrams to 3600 mg a day. This wide range of dosing makes it possible to slowly increase the medicine to achieve the desired effect while being able to minimize the side effects. Overall, gabapentin has been tremendously effective in treating nerve associated pain syndromes. Recently concerns have been rising about the street use of gabapentin mixed with other drugs, and an increase in death rates of individuals who mix gabapentin with opiates.

Pregabalin

Pregabalin (trade name Lyrica) is a chemical relative of gabapentin. It also works by binding to a subunit of the calcium ion channel proteins. Thus, we see a similar effect with inhibiting excitatory signals to the post-synaptic neuron, and therefore a decrease in the intensity of pain signals passing through the nervous system. It is relatively new in the marketplace, and shows great promise for chronic conditions associated with nerve pain.

Currently, pregabalin has indications for diabetic nerve pain, spinal injury associated pain, pain from shingles, fibromyalgia pain, and for the treatment of partial seizures.

Milnacipran

Milnacipran (trade name Savella) works by inhibiting serotonin and norepinephrine reuptake (similar to SNRIs). It is indicated in treating fibromyalgia. Initially it appeared to be extremely effective, but my experience is the pain relief from it slowly diminishes over time for a number of patients. This is terribly unfortunate, because many people who are clumped into that large category of fibromyalgia are often dependent on opiates, as few other medications provide long-term relief. Yet, it is certainly a viable alternative for some patients who suffer from fibromyalgia pain.

Ropinirole

Ropinirole (trade name Requip) and pramipexole (trade name Mirapex) stimulate dopamine receptors. Naturally, a concern would be its addiction potential, euphoric effects, etc. However, this does not seem to be an issue with this drug. Ropinirole and pramipexole are indicated for Parkinson's Disease and restless leg syndrome. Restless leg syndrome often brings pain and discomfort with the restless legs, and both of these medications provide relief. The benefits of these drugs have more to do with their effect in the tissues of the body outside of the brain, as dopamine is not only in our brain reward system, but is also key to our body's basic motor functions.

Acetaminophen

Acetaminophen comes in many names and formulations. It is most commonly known as Tylenol. This medication has a broad range of therapeutic effects and has many benefits, ranging from fever reduction to pain relief. Acetaminophen acts directly in the hypothalamus of the brain for fever control. The means of pain relief is not totally clear. This has been a safe standby for years, for all age ranges, with no risk of addiction, tolerance, or dependence.

The past few years we have seen much media coverage regarding the dangers of acetaminophen and there are a few risks which should be understood. It is largely metabolized in the liver, so high doses of the chemical can cause liver damage. Thus, we often see suicide attempts by taking massive doses of acetaminophen. Most adults can safely metabolize over 3 grams of acetaminophen daily, even over long periods of time, without any toxicity to the liver.

The exception to this is people who have renal impairment. Some of the products of the liver metabolism are then removed from the body through the kidneys. Anyone who has poor kidney function cannot remove these metabolic products, and can therefore build up a toxicity to the metabolites of acetaminophen. So, anyone with liver damage or kidney damage should not use acetaminophen, or do so only under the direction of a physician or pharmacist.

Worth noting is the combination of acetaminophen with many other compounds. It is very widely used in combination with opiates, as the combination seems to enhance the pain relief of the opiate, therefore requiring a lower opiate dose. This has been very beneficial in reducing the opiate load while maintaining pain control.

Here, I will wave a red flag. Those who abuse opiates often combine them with alcohol, which is even more hazardous if the opiate also contains acetaminophen. Alcohol is metabolized by the liver, and damages the liver. The combination of alcohol and acetaminophen is dangerous, greatly enhancing the potential damage to the liver. Individuals who have used alcohol chronically also

COMMON NSAIDS IN U.S.

Generic	Brand
celecoxib	Celebrex
diclofenac	Voltaren Gel
	Voltaire, Voltaire-XR
	Cataflam
	Cambia
	Zipsor
	Flector
	Pennsaid
etodolac	Lodine
fenoprofen	Nalfon
flurbiprofen	Ansaid
Ibuprofen	Caldolor
	Advil, Advil Migraine
	Motrin, Motrin IB
Indomethacin	Indocin
ketoprofen	
ketorolac	Sprix
	Toradol
meclofenamate	
mefenamic acid	Ponstel
meloxicam	Mobic
nabumetone	Relafen
naproxen	Anaprox, Anaprox DS
	EC-Naprosyn
	Naprelan
	Naprosyn
	Aleve
	Midol
	Pamprin
oxaprozin	Daypro
piroxicam	Feldene
sulindac	
tolmetin	

have to be careful when using acetaminophen, as they may have some liver damage already.

A number of products containing acetaminophen have recently been pulled off the market. This is due in large part to the excessive use of those products, beyond the recommendations for safe dosing. When used properly, acetaminophen has a very safe record as an effective pain reliever for most people.

Non-Steroidal Anti-Inflammatory Drugs (NSAIDs)

There are many NSAIDs available, both over the counter and prescription. These medications are potent pain relievers, very effective for controlling fevers, and in reducing inflammation (something that acetaminophen does not do). We see them used often for pain relief, and for inflammatory disorders.

Generally, NSAIDs are well tolerated. The most immediate danger is they reduce prostaglandin production, and prostaglandins are partially responsible for protecting the stomach from the intense acidic environment required to digest foods. Therefore, NSAID use can contribute to the development of ulcers.

In recent years, several variations of the NSAIDs have been developed. A class known as Cox-II inhibitors came to market. Some were pulled because of increased risk of heart problems, but others are still available, having shown no increase in risk of heart problems. General cautions to keep in mind, is anyone with known heart disease should not take NSAIDs, and elderly people tend to have a greater risk of side effects than a younger person.

COMBINATION NSAIDS

Chemical Name	Brand Name
naproxen/esomeprazole	Vimovo
diclofenac/misoprostol	Arthritic
ibuprofen/famotidine	Duexis
naproxen/sumatriptain	Treximet

Long-term use of NSAIDs can potentially damage the kidneys,

and as with any medication, there are other potential side effects. But for short-term relief of pain, used carefully, under proper dosing and guidelines NSAID's are safe and effective.

Treatments for Opiate Addiction

1. Naltrexone

A chemical that triggers a receptor is called an agonist. A chemical that blocks a receptor is called an antagonist. All the opiates/opioids discussed above, which can potentially lead to tolerance, abuse, and addiction, are opiate receptor agonists. There are several chemicals that block opiate receptors (naltrexone and naloxone) and have found to be effective in the treatment of opiate addiction.

2. Buprenorphine

One semi-synthetic opiate called buprenorphine is a partial agonist and partial antagonist. It is manufactured in several different forms that work well for addiction treatment and is now widely used for detoxification, and for long-term dependence during opiate treatment. One formulation is indicated for pain management, with a theoretical decreased risk of abuse.

These are very promising treatment options, though the government has limited the use of buprenorphine for the treatment of opiate addiction. Physicians are required to take a training class and obtain a special license to use this drug. Even then, they are limited to treating 300 patients at a time. This is to prevent diversion of the medication to the streets, as buprenorphine is popular to help street users through withdrawal from opiate abuse. Negatively, these restrictions severely limit the number of patients who can be treated for opiate addiction with this drug. And as with any new drug on the market, buprenorphine is quite expensive in any of its forms.

One brand name of buprenorphine is Suboxone. The Suboxone web site has a list of doctors in each state that are licensed to prescribe Suboxone or buprenorphine to opiate-dependent patients. This is not to be confused with another brand called Subutex. This pill only contains buprenorphine, and without the naloxone component, this drug is much easier to abuse and use incorrectly. These are called "subs" on the street.

The introduction of buprenorphine revolutionized the treatment of acute opiate withdrawal. Before this drug, we simply treated patients supportively for their symptoms, using medicines for the nausea, abdominal

OPIATE AGONISTS

Generic	Brand
Naltrexone	ReVia
	Vivitrol
Naloxone	Narcan

MIXED AGONISTS/ANTAGONISTS

Generic	Brand
Buprenorphine	Buprenex
	Subutex
	Butrans Transdermal
	Probuphine
Buprenorphine/ naloxone	Suboxone
	Zubsolv
	Bunavail

cramping, diarrhea, leg cramps, anxiety, pain, etc. There were many different combinations and tricks to help through the terrible opiate withdrawals.

3. Butrans

Butrans is the name for buprenorphine that comes in a patch. This is used for treatment of patients who have chronic low to moderate levels of pain. There is not a limit on the medical provider as to the number of patients they can treat with Butrans. Butrans is only approved for the treatment of pain, not for opiate addiction.

4. Vivitrol

Vivitrol is the brand name of naltrexone opiate blocker in an injectable form. It persists for 30 days in the tissues, and blocks the opiate receptors, being a pure antagonist. This has no risk for abuse. It prevents opiate effects, even if opiates are taken. There also appears to be a more rapid rebuilding of the body's own opiate system with the use of naltrexone. Studies show a decrease in cravings for opiates with the use of Vivitrol during recovery treatment. Any doctor can prescribe this, but most are not comfortable doing so, as its broad use is relatively new, and it is used in a select group of patients. Unfortunately, it is also very expensive.

5. Methadone

Methadone is used for the treatment of heroin addiction, as well as opiate addiction or dependence in general. The reasoning for using methadone even though it is a full opiate agonist and addictive, is because it is easier to control than heroin. Heroin use resulted in such a high death rate from overdose that the medical community wanted anything to stop the devastation. Methadone did indeed reduce the death rates from street opiate overdose, particularly heroin. Like other opiates, methadone leads to worse dependence, tolerance, and increasing doses. The drug also has some long-lasting and toxic metabolic products that some people do not tolerate, and can be dangerous. When Methadone clinics first popped up, patients had to go in daily for their dose of methadone. Clinic models have changed since then. Some places dispense several days' worth of methadone if the patient shows stability and good behavior.

Methadone has been the recommended opiate to use during pregnancy in the past. An opiate addicted mother should not abruptly stop her opiates, as opiate withdrawal can be harmful to a fetus. To control the opiate use, methadone has been substituted for other opiates, and then the newborn treated for opiate withdrawal. Even this, however, is changing. Studies are being done with buprenorphine that show it may be preferable to methadone. Buprenorphine is revolutionizing treatment for opiates. Much of the methadone business is giving way to buprenorphine treatment. However, the limited availability of buprenorphine makes this change a slow and difficult process. Buprenorphine may not be the ideal form of treatment, but it is much safer, and unlike methadone, buprenorphine appears to decrease the dependence on opiates over time.

APPENDIX E

BENZODIAZEPINES

Benzodiazepines (benzos) were developed in the late 1950's, and came to market in the early 1960's. They work for sedation, anxiety, muscle relaxation, insomnia, and treating seizures. Because of an improved safety profile, they quickly replaced barbiturates, except for certain applications in anesthesia and for some seizure conditions, barbiturates became a drug of the past.

Well-known brand names of benzos are Xanax, Valium, and Ativan. The list here shows the more common benzodiazepines used in the United States, as well as worldwide. Some of the most popular drugs being used for anxiety disorders are alprazolam, diazepam, and clonazepam. Severe muscle injuries not responsive to other muscle relaxants respond very well to diazepam. Diazepam and chlordiazepoxide also work together to prevent Delirium Tremens and seizures during alcohol withdrawal. Many of the benzos are used as effective sleep aids. Others, such as midazolam are used for sedation during procedures, with the added benefit of amnesia. Patients given this drug often do not remember the procedure.

Despite being much safer than the barbiturates, benzodiazepines still have potential drawbacks. Most benzodiazepines are indicated for short-term use only. If used frequently, or long-term, the body can build a tolerance to them, and grow dependent on them. When benzos are used for months or years, and the individual using them cannot safely stop them without significant and potentially dangerous withdrawal, with dramatically worse symptoms than when they started using the drug.

What usually happens is a low dose benzo may work wonderfully for anxiety or insomnia to begin with, but neither of those conditions generally resolves within a week or two. After a couple of months of using the medicine, it just doesn't seem to work anymore. The dose is then gently increased, and again it works very well until it doesn't, and this vicious cycle repeats. Over time, the patient becomes dependent on a large dose of the benzos, and yet no longer benefits from the drug, but cannot stop it without potentially having a seizure. They cannot taper down the dosage without suffering more severe anxiety or insomnia than before they ever started the medicine.

They simply cannot stop on their own, but are sick of taking a medicine which no longer works. This is often the point at which patients seek treatment for "addiction", which in this case is actually drug dependence, unless they have abused the benzo (in which case it then qualifies as addiction).

The risk of tolerance, dependence, and abuse is often related to the duration of action of a

COMMON BENZODIAZEPINES

Generic	Brand
alprazolam	Xanax
	Xanax XR
	Niravam
chlordiazepoxide	Librium
clobazam	Onfi
clonazepam	Klonopin
clorazepate	Tranxene SD
	Tranxene T-Tab
diazepam	Valium
	Diazepam Auto-Injector
estazolam	
flurazepam	Dalmane
flunitrazepam	Rohypnol (illegal in US)
lorazepam	Ativan
midazolam	Versed
oxazepam	Serax
temazepam	Restoril
triazolam	Halcion

BENZODIAZEPINE-LIKE MEDICATIONS

eszopiclone	Lunesta
zaleplon	Sonata
zolpidem	Ambien

BENZODIAZEPINE BLOCKER

flumazenil	Romazicon

drug. In other words, in dealing with potentially addictive substances, shorter acting medications are more addictive. The frequency of dosing of a medicine is usually a good indicator of its addictive potential. Dosing of a drug is generally done based on the half-life of the drug. A drug's half-life is the time which it takes your system to remove one-half of the medicine from the body.

Most drugs have to be repeated before the time of the half-life in order to maintain a therapeutic effect. For example, alprazolam is a short-acting benzo and has a half-life of about 11 hours. It is recommended to be dosed every 8 hours, but is often given every 6 hours because the effect begins to wear off. Clonazepam, on the other hand, is a long acting benzo, and has a 20-hour half-life. It works well when dosed every 12 hours, though it can be used every 8 hours.

The onset of action of the drug is also reflective of the duration of the drug. Alprazolam has a very rapid onset of action, and is thus preferred by those who are having a severe anxiety attack. Clonazepam, on the other hand, takes twenty to thirty minutes to begin to work, and is thus less popular for those who suffer acute anxiety.

All of these characteristics add to the complexity of addiction potential. More rapid acting and short acting drugs seem to develop a tolerance more quickly. Thus, a benzo or a pain medicine that must be used every four to six hours is much more likely to induce a tolerance, dependence, and ultimately has a greater potential for addiction.

The rapid onset of a drug also seems to be more likely to induce a state of mild euphoria. With the benzodiazepines, the euphoria felt is a well-being that possibly is better than the person's normal sensation of well-being. When the benzo wears off, the user returns to a state of normal, which to them now seems subnormal. The complete absence of anxiety during the initial rush of the drug makes the user's normal life, with its inherent and ever-present life stressors, seem like they are returning back into a state of anxiety. This often precipitates another anxiety attack. The anxiety in turn induces the user to want to take another dose of the drug, returning them to a fairytale state of anxiety-free living. This is one of the mechanisms of drug dependence and addiction to benzodiazepines.

This state of carefree living seems to be a common theme amongst drug users, and is often the desired effect we see in abuse of such substances as opiates and marijuana. Unfortunately, once the drug is no longer used or cannot be obtained, the end result is a constant state of fear, pain, or anxiety. Over time, the drug no longer works as well to produce the same carefree state. The relentless longing to live in that condition, along with the ever-increasing dread of facing the normal stresses of life (that now seem monstrous and insurmountable) leads to combining drugs and the quest to find the right drug cocktail to regain their sense of well-being.

Drug cocktails become more common as the duration of drug use prolongs. Certainly, some addicts combine drugs simply to see how high they can push their high, but it doesn't take long for a drug user to fall into the pattern of use to avoid withdrawal, or to try to feel normal and be able to function.

STREET NAMES [1, 2, 3]

BZDs
Benzos
Downers
Goofballs
Heavenly Blues
Qual
Orbital
Stupefy
Tranx
Tranks
Nerve Pills
Valley Girl
Xannies

Benzodiazepines make particularly effective, and dangerous, cocktails. As mentioned in the previous chapter, they can be mixed with barbiturates. The barbiturate not only has an addictive effect with the benzo, but they also enhance the receptor activity of the benzo receptors, amplifying the effect of the benzo. This is a very dangerous combination, making what would normally be a small dose of a benzo into a potentially life-threatening overdose. Similar cocktails with deadly risks are seen when mixing benzos with alcohol, opiates, and other drugs. There is really no limit to the combination of illicit and prescription drugs that have been taken to increase the high, reduce the withdrawals, minimize anxiety, or treat other symptoms seen with frequent drug use. Even mixing long, medium, and short acting benzos to gain a faster, yet longer duration of relief from symptoms is commonplace.

Benzodiazepines are frequently implicated in overdose deaths, but when investigated, it rarely turns out that the person who died used a benzo in isolation. Overdose deaths by pure benzodiazepine use are relatively rare, but common when one or more other substances are used.

The tragedy about dependency on benzos is the circumstances leading to the use or abuse of the drug is rarely ever made better, and in most cases made worse by using the drug. Blog after blog can be read discussing how terrible a person's anxiety or insomnia is. They just cannot understand why the benzos have worked for years, but aren't working now. Meth addicts write how benzos solved their anxiety problems for so long, but their massive dose of xannies (Xanax) doesn't do it anymore. They write how their Xanax barely maintains control if they stay on their prescription dose, and they have to take an extra pill so they can actually have a relaxing day.

To compound their problems, there is simply no other non-addictive drug that will relieve anxiety and insomnia as quickly and completely as a benzodiazepine. That is the danger of these

BENZODIAZEPINE EFFECTS

Short term:

Sedation
Anxiolytics
Anticonvulsants
Muscle relaxation
Respiratory depression
Amnesia
Anesthesia adjunct

Long term

Depression
Anxiety
Dependence
Cognitive defects

Paradoxical Effects

Aggression
Violence
Anxiety
Suicidality
Impulsivity
Abnormal behaviors
Poor social control

drugs. There are many other medicines which will help with anxiety, but they just do not make people feel as instantly good as the benzodiazepines. There are many other medicines which help with sleep, but they do not work as well in providing immediate and restorative sleep as do the benzos.

Interestingly, one of the most effective methods of reducing anxiety is to employ counseling and bio-feedback techniques. But most people do not want to put forth the time and effort to apply these methods. They want an instant fix, for anxiety is terrifying.

Having explained all this, it is safe to say benzodiazepines do have a place in medical practice. They work on the GABA receptor, thus removing some inhibitions and causing relaxation in the mammalian system. Legitimate and effective uses include sedation, anesthesia, breaking acute anxiety attacks (which can be dangerous and may escalate if not monitored closely), stopping or preventing seizures, relaxing spastic muscles, inducing sleep in severely sleep-deprived individuals, and more.

Long-term treatment for seizures with some benzos has shown to be safe with little chance of dose escalation if the benzo is used correctly. Benzodiazepines are also wonderful aids in emergency situations to resolve agitation associated with trauma, anxiety produced by life-threatening conditions such as a heart attack, or relieving the agitation from drug overdose and drug withdrawal. We even use them to keep patient's safe and more comfortable during the acute withdrawal of alcohol, despite those individuals being more prone to addiction. The risk of using benzos to acutely withdraw an individual from alcohol is very minimal.

Benzodiazepines must be used with much caution in children and senior citizens. The negative effects in children is, again, the potential for direct impact on the development of the prefrontal cortex, and thus, the ability to make decisions and understand consequences. In older people, the metabolism is slowed, and the effects and side effects are amplified. This is especially true when the medicine has an active metabolite, and the concentration of the active substance builds up in the system of an individual because the person cannot break it down as quickly as it is being taken.

Pregnancy is an absolute no for the use of benzodiazepines if there are any possible alternatives, as the fetus can become addicted. There is also a possible link between cleft palate and benzo use during pregnancy, though this is still not well established.

In rare cases, there are patients who have been on a low-dose benzo for twenty to thirty years, never escalating the dose, and still benefiting from the effect of the medicine. This is an exception to the rule. Addiction is a universal danger of benzos, even when prescribed by a physician.

Tips for the safe use of benzodiazepines:

1. If using for sleep or anxiety, never use more than 2-3 weeks.
2. Look for any other means of treating the condition you have, even if it seems slightly less effective, particularly for anxiety and insomnia.
3. Take the medication as prescribed by the doctor. Do not take more than prescribed, and be aware many doctors are not trained in addiction. Because of this, they may not realize the risk, or know how to help if you become dependent on the medicine.
4. Never mix benzodiazepines with other sedating medications or substances, especially alcohol.
5. If you are taking a benzodiazepine and find it is no longer working well, or you are having to increase your dose, talk to your physician immediately (or find one who is willing to discuss this with you) about tapering you off the benzo, while helping you find a safer alternative. Do not stop it abruptly, especially if you are on a high dose or have taken it for a long time. Sudden benzodiazepine withdrawal can cause seizures.

BENZODIAZEPINE WITHDRAWAL

anxiety
mood swings
depersonalization
insomnia
nausea and vomiting
confusion
loss of memory
headache
pain
social isolation
fatigue
hallucinations
seizures
psychosis
suicidality
headaches
tremor
weight loss
depression
intense sweating
irritability
panic attacks
risk of falls
neurologic impairment
death

ALTERNATIVES TO BENZOS

NON-BENZODIAZEPINE MUSCLE RELAXERS:

Carisoprodol

Having concluded our discussion of benzodiazepines, I feel it is important to discuss a medicine called carisoprodol, also marketed as Soma. This medicine is marketed as a muscle relaxer, and is not a controlled substance. Many people take this medicine for pain, particularly for muscle pain.

Carisoprodol is metabolized into meprobamate, which is an older anxiolytic. The references for the medications explain that it is a non-benzodiazepine anxiolytic, but the exact mechanism of action is unknown. This does not prove anything terrible about the medication. However, as I have practiced addiction medicine, I have seen individuals who were dependent on carisoprodol. The drug also carries warnings about seizures if abruptly stopping the medicine after long-term use. I have seen a seizure after someone stopped carisoprodol, and I now use medication to prevent seizures in people withdrawing from carisoprodol just as I would from a benzodiazepine.

Meprobamate drug information says there is evidence for risk to a human fetus if used during pregnancy, and is listed as a Category D. Carisoprodol is listed as Category C, meaning there has been evidence for harm in animal fetuses, but no tests have been done in humans.

Methocarbamol

There are several other "muscle relaxants" which are used for spasm and muscle pain. These are sometimes given for restless leg syndrome, and anything which may include muscle cramping or pain, including withdrawal from opiates and other drugs of abuse. Methocarbamol is one such medicine, also marketed as Robaxin. It is safe and effective if taken for the proper reason, under proper dosages.

The mechanism of action is unknown, but it works by depressing the central nervous system (CNS). This results in a sedative effect, and therefore is dangerous to use in combination with other CNS depressants. Methocarbamol is unfortunately becoming a popular street drug, even though it has very low addictive potential. The sedation effect seems to be sought after. It provides ease from muscle cramps during withdrawal. It also helps inmates sleep away their time, so it is often sought after by people in jail.

Cyclobenzaprine

Marketed also as Flexeril, cyclobenzaprine is another muscle relaxant that is centrally acting. Again, its mechanism of action is not known exactly, though it does enhance norepinephrine, and binds to serotonin receptors, and is similar to the old tri-cyclic antidepressants. It is an effective muscle relaxant with low potential for addiction. But if used at high doses for extended periods can cause an uncomfortable withdrawal.

There is a street value for cyclobenzaprine, though less than methocarbamol, and its use seems to be more regionalized than methocarbamol. It is crushed and used on the streets as "mellow yellow" or "cyclone." Taken in large doses it gives a mellow sense of pleasure, but can be dangerous if taken in high doses. The drug suppresses the central nervous system, producing drowsiness as well as slowing the heart rate and the respirations.

It too can be combined with other drugs to enhance CNS depression, and the mind-altering effects of those drugs. Cyclobenzaprine is becoming a popular method of enhancing the effects of opiates. It potentiates the opiates, making the euphoria produced stronger. Taken in high doses it can cause convulsions, severe drowsiness, irregular heartbeat, hallucinations, change in body temperature, nervousness, nausea, and vomiting. Taken as directed for indicated uses, it is a safe and effective medication.

Tizanidine

Tizanidine is another muscle relaxant. It works by increasing the inhibition of the pre-synaptic motor neurons and reducing the spasticity of muscle. It is marketed as Zanaflex. Thus far, I have seen little tendency towards abuse of this medicine aside from the individual who takes high doses in an attempt to get high. Many have reported it is the most effective pain relief they have had relative to muscle spasm, in conjunction with their regular pain medicine. As with any medicine, it is abusable, but there seem to be less effects from it that would lead to abuse than with the other muscle relaxants.

Non-benzodiazepine anxiolytics:

Hydroxyzine

This medicine is an antihistamine. It is also marketed under the trade names Vistaril and Atarax. It has a broad range of antihistamine effects, including anti-itch, anti-rash, etc. As with most of the older antihistamines, it is potentially sedating, and this sedation probably accounts for the anti-anxiety effect produced. It has very little abuse potential.

Hydroxyzine does pass into the brain. Because of this, it has the effects of sedation, anti-anxiety, and even has some anti-psychotic effects. It reduces nausea, dizziness, and aids with motion sickness.

As an anxiolytic, hydroxyzine has become very useful. It is an effective alternative for the barbiturates and benzodiazepines, and is very helpful during acute withdrawal and acute abstinence syndromes after stopping many of the drugs of abuse. As mentioned previously, insomnia and anxiety are common complaints with drug abusers. Hydroxyzine is a safe and effective means of dealing with both types of symptoms. It does not give the euphoric sense of well-being, and thus is often felt to be less effective for reducing anxiety, because it does not cause the euphoric relaxation produced by the benzos.

Hydroxyzine has been found to enhance the effects of opiates. This makes it a useful medication for pain control. However, drug abusers have discovered this, and use it to increase the effects of opiates. Therefore, it is still abused on the streets to enhance opiate effects, even though hydroxyzine itself has very little addictive potential.

Buspirone

Buspirone is another medication well suited to treat anxiety disorders. The brand name is BuSpar. It is quite different in structure and function than the benzos and barbiturates, yet still very effective for anxiety disorders. It works on the serotonin receptors; thus it has similar effects to the antidepressants that work on serotonin along with its anti-anxiety properties. It also works on the dopamine receptors. But, despite having dopamine activity, buspirone has not shown any pattern of addiction or dependence after prolonged use.

Buspirone works well for the acute and post-acute anxiety of drug use. It does not protect from the dangers of withdrawal from benzos, barbiturates, or alcohol, but it is quite effective in controlling the anxiety produced by those drugs. Again, it does not cause the euphoric feelings of those drugs, and so many addicts do not feel it is as effective. Buspirone also takes longer to start working, and can be taken on a schedule in order to get the anxiolytic effects.

Blogs by abusers generally throw buspirone out as a potentially abusable drug. There is very little of the effect from it which addicts desire. There are many potential side-effects if used in higher doses, though.

Antidepressants

There are many medications which affect serotonin uptake. These include selective serotonin re-uptake inhibitors (SSRIs) and serotonin/norephineprine re-uptake inhibitors (SNRIs). In my experience, the SNRI's have been a little more effective as anxiolytics, though both classes have distinct, desired results on reducing anxiety. Specific drugs within each class seem to work better than other drugs in the same class, and often it seems that a person's individual genetic characteristics determines the effectiveness of which drug will work the best for them.

These medications are generally known as anti-depressants. Some have been around for a very long time, and are well known. Many people are afraid of this class of drugs, and many people tell me they do not want to take them because they have heard they are addicting.

These medications are not addicting by the definition of addiction. I have never yet met someone who has taken an antidepressant to get high, or has increasingly abused the drug for the sake of euphoria.

The confusion probably arises because of the effect of the medicines, and what happens if they are abruptly stopped. If we consider how they work, we see that they enhance the effect of serotonin and norepinephrine in the brain, keeping those two neurotransmitters in the nerve synapses for longer periods of time. These are potent neurotransmitters. If we enhance them, and suddenly remove them, the person who was taking them will experience symptoms of serotonin or norepinephrine deprivation.

This leads to the common misconception that they are addicting, and have withdrawal syndromes associated with their use. Any such "withdrawal" or abstinence syndrome can be avoided by tapering their use over several weeks, allowing the body to adjust to the decrease in the serotonin or norepinephrine. This is really no different than the need to slowly increase the dose when starting the medications to minimize the risk of side effects.

Bupropion (commonly known as Wellbutrin) has a different mechanism of action. It is often lumped into this category because it is an effective antidepressant. It inhibits norepinephrine and dopamine uptake. However, in my experience, it has very little benefit in reducing anxiety. It is often combined with an SSRI to help with the depression while utilizing the SSRI for the anxiety component.

Antidepressants have certainly been abused in attempts to get a buzz or a high. However, most addicts say they are wasting their time trying to get anything from an antidepressant. The reality is that using these medicines in high doses can cause a very dangerous condition called Serotonin Syndrome. Rather than a high or euphoria, they become very sick. Thus, SSRIs and SNRIs are quite safe at prescribed doses, and quite effective for treating anxiety.

Once again, however, these medications may take several weeks to produce their effect, having to build up to a certain level of serotonin or norepinephrine within the brain to work. In addition, they are generally started at a low dose to avoid side effects, and may have to be slowly increased over weeks or months to become effective. Thus, someone who is suffering from acute anxiety syndrome often decides these medicines do not work at all, and quits taking them before they have a chance to work.

This "failure" can often be alleviated by using different medicines in combination, for their strengths. For example, using a short-acting medicine such as hydroxyzine or buspirone for acute anxiety attacks for the first month or two while waiting for an SSRI or SNRI to become effective is quite safe. This can even be safely done using a benzodiazepine short term (two weeks) while waiting for the antidepressant to begin working as an anxiolytic. Obviously, however, the benzo combination should never be used in someone who has abusive tendencies or who has ever abused benzos. One should also be aware that even after short-term use of any benzo, certain individuals will feel there is nothing else that alleviates their anxiety adequately.

APPENDIX F

Sedative Hypnotics and Sleepers

Classifying certain drugs into categories can be difficult. Sedative hypnotics can refer to many kinds of drugs. Any drug that has sedating qualities could be considered one of this class. I have chosen to include only certain sleeping aids in this chapter. Benzodiazepines are also classified as sedative hypnotics, as are barbiturates. However, they warrant their own chapters, for the sake of understanding their own particularly unique risks and benefits.

This chapter will explore many different sleep aids. Originally the intent was to review the addictive nature of commonly used medications. However, there are some medications which can be very useful and safe. Therefore, further discussion is needed to make clear that not all sleep aids are addictive.

This will not be all inclusive, nor will it address herbal or natural supplements to any significant extent, as those are beyond the scope of this reference. It will attempt to review the medications which have been FDA approved as sleep aids. This, in hopes of giving some viable options and warning of dangers, while providing tools to help recovering addicts through the tough times of early sobriety.

Before embarking on a discussion of sleep aids, we must discuss insomnia. Insomnia and anxiety are the two most common long term physical side effects that I see in those recovering from chronic drug abuse. Sleep patterns are terribly disrupted during drug abuse and addiction. There are many reasons for this, including psychological stress, physical habituation, emotional dependence, etc. There is no immediate cure, no magic pill. Yet the vast majority of people who are coming off drugs want a magic pill to fix their sleep. Sleep deprivation is devastating to the immune system, to the psyche, and to the spirit. The need for sleep becomes an overwhelming drive for the recovering addict. Sleep deprivation alone drives many to relapse to their drug use.

Insomnia is also a terrible problem for many people who have never experienced addiction. Tremendous research on sleep has given us a growing advantage on sleep disorders and how to deal with them. The development of medications to help with sleep is one of the direct results of that research. Besides medications, the internet is filled with information on sleep hygiene. These sites are some of the best resources for those with insomnia. Sleep hygiene can be a very effective tool to restore sleep. Full spectrum lighting can also contribute to sleep pattern restoration. However, reconditioning our mind and body to healthy sleep patterns requires patience and persistence. Just as the sleep disorder took years to develop, so it may take years to correct.

Sleep is controlled largely by our body's Circadian Rhythm—a cycle of wakefulness and sleepiness that occurs on a twenty-four hour cycle. The rhythm is driven by light (and can be upset and altered by electric lights). Light enters our eyes, where special photosensitive cells transmit a signal to the hypothalamus which then signals the pineal gland. The pineal gland controls the release of melatonin, adjusts body temperature, and influences the release of cortisol in the blood. These factors are the major players in the sleep/wake cycle. Therefore, we can see that while sedation may assist in a person going to sleep, it will not correct sleep cycles or sleep patterns. There is much more involved. Sleep medications, then, are only tools to assist in adjusting those sleep cycles by inducing sleep. Other measures to slowly change the body cycle and chemistry must be put in place with the medications, or they are ineffective for long term change.

A. Benzodiazepine-like medications:

Benzodiazepines are good for inducing a close to normal sleep. Whereas some medications just induce drowsiness and leave one feeling drugged, benzodiazepines seem to induce a restful and restorative sleep. However, because of the potential for dependence, abuse, and addiction, other medications were developed. This "non-benzodiazepine" class of medications interact with the GABA-benzodiazepine receptors. Thus, we should expect a very benzodiazepine-like effect.

BENZODIAZEPINE-LIKE MEDICATIONS

Generic	Brand
eszopiclone	Lunesta
zaleplon	Sonata
zolpidem	Ambien
	Ambien CR
	Edluar
	Intermezzo
	Zolpimist

This is exactly what we do see. With the exception of eszopiclone (marketed as Lunesta), they are only recommended for short term use. This is because they can still be habit forming, and then one is unable to sleep without the medication anyway. Interestingly, eszopiclone has not shown dependence with extended use.

Zolpidem (best known as Ambien) is a very common and a very requested sleeping aid. However, as with so many other of the addictive drugs, in some people zolpidem causes dependence, tolerance, and escalation of dose to maintain the sedative effect. Because of this it is often abused. It is also gaining a reputation for causing people to do things which they do not remember doing, along with causing hallucinations and other undesirable side effects. I have had several patients who have no recollection of things they did during the night, such as going out for walks, making phone calls, and eating. Some have awakened to find themselves in strange places, in different or no clothing, quite disturbed by what had happened that they could not remember.

Many people depend on alcohol to sleep. Often, they combine sedatives with the alcohol, which becomes a very dangerous cocktail. Mixing of such drugs is, unfortunately, the cause of many overdoses.

These medications are effective sleep aids. However, the use of either zolpidem or zaleplon

BENZODIAZEPINES COMMONLY USED FOR SLEEP

Generic	Brand
estazolam	
flurazepam	Dalmane
lorazepam	Ativan
temazepam	Restoril
triazolam	Halcion

BARBITURATES USED FOR SLEEP

Generic	Brand
Butabarbital	Butisol
Secobarbital	Seconal

ANTIHISTAMINES

Generic	Brand
doxylamine	Unisom Sleep Tabs
hydroxyzine	Mistral
	Atarax
diphenhydramine	Nytol
	Simply Sleep
	Sominex Maximum Strength
	Sominex Original
	Tranquil
	Unisom SleepGels,
	Unisom SleepMelts,
	Unisom SleepTabs
	Vicks ZzzQuil

should be limited to a maximum of two weeks, and only as an adjunct to restoring a normal sleep cycle. The underlying concept of sleep restoration should revolve around resetting the sleep cycle.

B. Benzodiazepines

As noted previously, benzodiazepines have an entire chapter dedicated to them. Nothing more will be explained here, other than giving reference to the names of commonly prescribed "sleepers" from the benzo class. See Appendix E

C. Barbiturates

Similarly, barbiturates have a dedicated chapter. See Appendix D.

D. Antihistamines

Most people are familiar with antihistamines. They are wonderful for inhibiting allergic reactions. Some of the more exciting breakthroughs in treating allergies in the past few decades have been the development of the "non-sedating" antihistamines. Benadryl (diphenhydramine) is one of the better-known antihistamines. It is well known for sedation also, and is commonly used as a sleep aid, such as with Tylenol PM, Simply Sleep, Unisom SleepGels, and others. Some cousins also make an appearance for sleep aids, such as doxylamine and hydroxyzine.

Antihistamines are also used to help motion sickness, nausea, and vertigo. They are wonderfully helpful for people who are ill from allergies, motion sickness, or inner ear problems. However, they are universally known for their side effects, and many people avoid them because they become too tired to function, or drowsy, dizzy, or impaired in coordination. This is one of the disadvantages of using them as sleep aids. They do help insomniacs fall asleep. However, often-times they wake up feeling somewhat sluggish or impaired. Antihistamines are rarely abused, probably because they do not cause euphoria, and there are other sedating drugs that feel much better, such as benzodiazepines.

E. Tricyclic AntidepressantsTricyclics

Tricyclic antidepressants are an older class of antidepressants. They are not used as much anymore due to undesirable side effects, one of which is sedation. Drowsiness is a common side effect. At smaller than normal doses, they are mildly sedating while avoiding some of the other undesirable side effects. These medications are very useful in treating individuals for insomnia while withdrawing from drugs, and seem especially effective during post-withdrawal insomnia for alcoholics. Trazodone is commonly and effectively used as a sleep aid. Perhaps some of the antidepressant characteristics are beneficial during this period of recovery. Though we do see people overdose on tricyclics, they do not seem to be addictive or habit forming.

TRICYCLIC ANTIDEPRESSANTS

Generic	Brand
trazodone	Oleptro
doxepin	Silenor

F. Antipsychotics

Quetiapine is an antipsychotic often used for bipolar disorder. It is quite sedating and so the dose is typically escalated rapidly to obtain the psychiatric effect while pushing through the sedation. However, maintained at a low dose it seems to give an antihistamine-like effect, with mild sedation that helps induce sleep. It is not, however, approved as a sleep aid, and such "off label" use of quetiapine is leading to street availability of the drug, along with attempts to abuse it. It is also being effectively used for behavioral problems arising from dementia, particularly related to anxiety.

Quetiapine has been used for acute opiate and cocaine withdrawals. It is also being studied for decreasing the cravings for cocaine. This medication is being studied for effectiveness in treating stimulant addiction, particularly when associated with psychiatric illness. However, the world of street prescription drug abuse leads to experimentation with anything available, and is often further ahead in finding abuse potential for drugs than the scientific data is in finding benefit.

Unfortunately, quetiapine is being abused on the streets. This may have several explanations. It seems to heighten the buzz associated with heroin, while easing the withdrawal from cocaine. Addicts who have been strung out for days without any sleep (such as with methamphetamine) find quetiapine to be very effective at inducing an immediate sleep, along with taking away symptoms of paranoia associated with use and withdrawal. Thus, it is finding its way into combinations with street drugs, and to ease the withdrawals from stimulants, or the drug deprivation symptoms between use. While it does not seem to cause a euphoria, it is

ANTIPSYCHOTICS

Generic	Brand
quetiapine	Seroquel

STREET NAMES FOR QUETIAPINE

Quells
Snoozeberries
Suzie-Qs
Q-Ball (combination of quetiapine with a speedball — which is the combination of heroin and cocaine)

abused for sedation, and inmates have reportedly complained of psychiatric symptoms in order to get quetiapine. Medication induced sedation is very popular amongst inmates, who will use any number of medicines such as muscle relaxers, antihistamines, and antipsychotics to help sleep away their jail time.

As with many of the other drugs that become both beneficial and detrimental in the world of abuse and addiction treatment, quetiapine's mechanism of action may explain why it is used. It does work on dopamine receptors in the brain, as do so many other of the abused drugs. It also has some effects on serotonin receptors. Again, this combination could make it very useful in treating addiction or dependence. Sadly, abuse leads to rapid discovery of effects while risking lives to do so. Studies are still working to find out exactly the risks and benefits of quetiapine in the setting of safe treatment.

G. Melatonin

MELATONIN

Many over the counter and herbal formulations

MELATONIN ENHANCING

Generic	Brand
ramelteon	Rozerem

A logical approach to repairing a damaged sleep cycle is to try and restore the body's natural sleep processes. Since melatonin is key to the sleep cycle, using melatonin to enhance sleep cycles makes sense. Many melatonin supplements are available, as well as a prescription medicine called ramelteon, which activates melatonin receptors.

A compelling study was performed by Dr. Mariangela Rondanelli, Ph.D. at the University of Pavia, Italy, in which patients were given melatonin along with zinc and magnesium supplements before bedtime for eight weeks. There was a significant improvement in the patients' sleep, and in how they felt during the day. [1]

It is important to emphasize that behaviors are key to sleep. Melatonin is naturally released by exposure to light (most effectively by sun light, but also by electric light), and taking melatonin to compensate or overcome natural light cycles is not going to be very effective. For this reason, sleep hygiene principles to modify sleep disorders, along with supplements that enhance or slightly modify the body's sleep cycle, promise to be the most effective in restoring natural sleep patterns.

APPENDIX G

Stimulants

Stimulants are a group of medicines that can be very useful on one hand, and very dangerous on the other. As a group, they are very commonly abused. Some of the more recognized stimulants include cocaine, amphetamine, methamphetamine, MDMA (ecstasy), nicotine, Ritalin, and caffeine. Prescription stimulants are readily available, and are thus also commonly abused drugs despite attempts to control the prescribing of these medications.

These medications increase alertness and capacity for performance, or the perceived capacity for improved performance. They are used by many people to gain a sudden increase in strength, speed, alertness, dexterity, mental processing, and overall enhancement of function. Needless to say, this has led to research and development in the area of stimulants for many years, from home applications to military applications. Efforts are still being made to find "safe" stimulants, meaning they have the effect of increasing performance and tolerance without causing the typical problems we see with performance improving stimulant use, such as heart failure, heart attacks, rebound anxiety, etc.

In contrast to the relatively low doses of caffeine we see in coffee and soft drinks, we have seen the additional physical risk of high doses of caffeine with the introduction of monster drinks, especially among teenagers. SAMSA reported increasing ER visits as a result of highly concentrated caffeine. As reported by NPR:

"The new numbers on emergency department visits come from the Substance Abuse and Mental Health

COMMON PRESCRIPTION AND OTC STIMULANTS

Chemical Names	Brand Names
armodafinil	Nuvigil
caffein	NoDoz
	ReCharge
	Vivarin
dexmethylphenidate	Focalin
	Focalin XR
dextroamphetamine	Dexedrine
	ProCentra
	Zenzedi
dextroamphetamine/ amphetamine	Adderall
	Adderall XR
lisdexamfetamine	Vyvanse
methamphetamine	Desoxyn
methylphenidate	Concerta
	Daytrana
	Metadate CD
	Metadate ER
	Methylin
	Methylin ER
	Quilivant XR
	Ritalin
	Ritalin LA
	Ritalin SR
modafinil	Provigil

NON-PRESCRIPTION STIMULANTS

cocaine
methamphetamine

STREET NAMES OF STIMULANTS [1,2,3]

R-ball	Crosses
Skippy	Hearts
The smart drug	LA turnaround
Vitamin R	Uppers
JIF	Bumblebees
Kibbles and bits	Pep Pills
Speed	Uppers
Truck Drivers	Co-Pilots
Bennies	Ups
Black beauties	

Methamphetamine

Ice, Speed, Crystal Meth, Crank, Crystal, Methadrine, Hearts, Bennies, Uppers, Amps, Pick me ups, Pickups

Cocaine

Nose Candy, Powder, Coke, Blow, BigC, Snow, White, Lady, Snowbirds, Cookie, Flake, Dust

Crack Cocaine

Kryptonite, Cookies, Strong

Services Administration, which tracks drug-related ER visits. They found that energy drink-related visits rose from 10,068 in 2007 to 20,783 in 2011. That's out of more than 1 million drug-related ER visits, the agency says. Before 2007, energy drink incidents were too few to report, the paper says.

"About 60 percent of the patients were seeking help with adverse reactions to the energy drink alone, while 27 percent had also taken prescription drugs. About 13 percent of patients had downed energy drinks and alcohol, and 10 percent had combined energy drinks and illegal drugs. Teenagers and young adults were most likely to end up in the ER.

"The face-palm stat: 9 percent of the unfortunates had combined energy drinks with prescription stimulants like Ritalin, giving them a double dose of chemical buzz." [4]

Certainly, the makers of the energy drinks contest the findings, and raise the concern that there may be other factors involved in the emergency room visits. However, it is simply common sense that such products could increase risks.

Can we extrapolate any lessons we learn from caffeine to other stimulants? Certainly! The mechanisms of action may differ, as well as the intensity of the effects, and of the side effects. The dangers are also relative to the potency and method of use of the drugs. Caffeine is, shall we say, one of the safest stimulants. However, it is still a stimulant, and can help us understand the effects of the more dangerous stimulants. To understand this better, see the graphs in Chapter 8, "Repeated Use and Seeking Normalcy.

Certainly, with the list of useful effects which stimulants have, it would make sense to apply them for our benefit. However, the risks are high. There are many dangers associated with stimulant use, especially at high doses, or in a prolonged manner of use. As our purpose is to discuss issues related to addiction, we will not so much debate the risks and benefits of stimulant use, as to simply try to understand why, from an addiction standpoint, stimulants can be extremely dangerous. We should note that in cases such as with attention deficit disorder (ADD) and other similar conditions, using a stimulant can be very beneficial and very safe.

The prescription stimulants, while certainly abusable, can be wonderful in helping people function normally in society. Conditions such as narcolepsy and attention deficit respond very well to the proper medicines. However, it is critical that great care is taken in diagnosing these conditions correctly before starting any stimulant type medication. As can be seen by the list of stimulant effects, it is conceivable that anyone could feel better by using such drugs, even if they do not qualify according to established diagnostic criteria. Therefore, a trial of medication to see if they help, without a careful evaluation and correct diagnosis, could be very detrimental in the long run.

Stimulants come in many forms. Here is a brief review of a few of the stimulants:

EFFECTS OF STIMULANTS

Short Term

During Use:	**After Use:**
improved attention	decreased attention
increased energy	fatigue
increased strength	weakness
increased heart rate	decreased performance
increased blood glucose	disturbed sleep
increased alertness	decreased stamina
increased stamina	depression
increased mobility	
increased mental arousal	
opening of airways	
increased dopamine	
increased norepinephrine	
euphoria	
elevation in blood pressure	
improved mood or sense of wellness	

STIMULANT WITHDRAWAL

Anxiety
Insomnia
Hypersomnia
Fatigue
Increased appetite
Vivid unpleasant dreams
Psychomotor agitation

Cocaine

Cocaine has been used for thousands of years, extracted by chewing the leaves of the coca plant. In the early 1900's it was purified and became a popular ingredient in tonics and elixirs. Cocaine use became very popular in the 1970s, and had a large cultural impact over the next two decades. It became such a large part of the 60–70's culture that it has come to be known by dozens of names, and found its way into music, poetry, and everyday language.

It is a very dangerous stimulant. It is also highly addictive. Cocaine blocks dopamine re-uptake in the nerve synapses, resulting in much higher concentrations of dopamine than normal. This is the source of the intense "high" experienced by cocaine users. It is also the cause of the rapid and intense tolerance, and high addictive potential. This is one of the drugs which accounts for the common description of "chasing the high." It is not uncommon for cocaine addicts to search for a way to find the high that they experienced the first time they used it, but can never get that again. For this reason, they frequently combine cocaine with other drugs, the

ADVERSE STIMULANT EFFECTS

Abstinence syndrome (being without)

Withdrawal
Apathy
Depression
Fatigue
Exhaustion

Effects of long or high dose use

Addiction
Hostility and aggression
Paranoia
Heart attacks
High blood pressure
Malignant hyperthermia
Heart arrhythmias
Sudden death
Psychosis
Depression
Mania
Stroke
Cardiomyopathy
Seizures
Anorexia
Headaches
Abdominal pain
Nausea and vomiting
Decreased libido
Sexual dysfunction
Restlessness
Paresthesias
Menstrual irregularities
Sweating
Tremor
Speech disturbance

most well-known combination being the "speedball," a mix of heroin and cocaine. This combination dramatically increases the risk of serious side effects. Many other substances are also combined with cocaine.

Cocaine is inhaled (snorted) through the nose or dissolved in water and injected directly into a vein. Absorption through the nose is very rapid, and produces a very potent high. However, injection into the blood stream is even faster, and more dangerous, delivering the drug almost immediately to the brain. Crack cocaine is cocaine that has been processed to form a hard crystal substance that can be heated and inhaled. The absorption through the lungs is also very rapid, though not quite as rapid as injection. Smoking or injecting produces an intense high that lasts about 5-15 minutes. Snorting is a less intense high, settling in more slowly, but lasts longer, about 15-30 minutes.

Snorting cocaine often damages the nasal tissues. Over time people develop bloody noses, allergy-like symptoms such as runny nose, loss of ability to smell, hoarseness, difficulty swallowing, and other complications. Injecting cocaine (or any drug) brings with it a large risk of infections, such as hepatitis and HIV, or bacterial infections in the skin and blood that can be disfiguring and life threatening. Even without sharing needles there is a high risk of bacterial infections.

Cocaine is available by prescription for medicinal purposes. It is carefully controlled because of the risks that go with it. Some doctors use the medicinal form of cocaine for anesthesia and to decrease blood supply to areas such as the nose, eyes, and throat during surgical procedures and to decrease blood flow, such as with bloody noses. It is very effective, and very safe if used properly. Aside from the select surgical applications noted above, cocaine has no useful medical purpose.

The effect of decreasing blood flow can be very dangerous when the drug is abused. In larger amounts cocaine can decrease blood flow to areas so much that tissue and organ damage can occur. Swallowing cocaine can decrease blood flow to the stomach or bowel to the point that sections of bowel can die or develop gangrene. Sudden surges of cocaine in the blood can cause heart vessels to constrict, decreasing blood flow. This, in combination with the increased blood pressure and pulse can lead to heart attacks and cardiac arrest.

Currently there are no medications approved for the treatment of cocaine addiction. Treatment is primarily behavioral and counseling. However, because of the high level of cocaine abuse, much research is going into the development of medications that will help prevent use, reduce cravings, and help treat the dangerous and harmful effects of cocaine. A vaccine is also being studied, which may be able to prevent the cocaine molecule from entering into the brain tissues. [6]

COCAINE EFFECTS

Euphoria
Addiction
Severe allergic reaction
Hypertension
Heart attack
Stroke
Dilated pupils
Tachycardia/arrhythmias
Ventricular fibrillation
Anorexia
Headaches
Nausea and vomiting
Abdominal pain
Respiratory arrest
Seizures
Congestive heart failure
Death
Anxiety
Irritability
Restlessness
Paranoia
Psychosis
Hallucinations
Hyperthermia
Muscle destruction
Loss of taste and smell
Abdominal pain

STREET NAMES OF COCAINE [5]

Bernie's Flakes
Big Bloke
Bernie's Gold Dust
Big Flake
Blanca
Crack
Flake
Gold Dust
Haven Dust
Have A Dust
Icing
Line
Pearl
Paradise White
Snow White
Snowcones
Sleigh Ride
White Powder
White Mosquito
All-American Drug
California Cornflakes
Dream
Double Bubble
Florida Snow
Gift-Of-The-Sun
Foo-Foo Dust
Foo Foo
Girlfriend
Gin
Gift-Of-The-Sun-God
Hunter
King's Habit
King
Love Affair
Late Night
Movie Star Drug
Pimp
Scorpion
Schoolboy
Sevenup
Studio Fuel
Star-Spangled Powder
Stardust
Society High
Burnese
Inca Message
Peruvian
Perico Cocaine
Percio
Percia
Peruvian Lady
Peruvian Flake
Bolivian Marching Powder
Big Rush
Bouncing Powder
Friskie Powder

STREET NAMES OF COCAINE *(continued)*

Glad Stuff
Happy Trails
Happy Powder
Happy Dust
Love Affair
Marching Powder
Marching Dust
Nose Powder
Nose Candy
Paradise
Nose Stuff
Aunt Nora
Angie
Bernie
Bernice
Billie Hoke
Cecil
Carrie Nation
Carrie
Choe
Chippy
Charlie
Corrinne
Corrine
Henry VIII
Her
Jejo
Lady Snow
Merck
Merk
Nieve
Mujer
Schmeck
Serpico 21
Scottie
C
Big C
C-Game
Coke
Coconut
Coca
Cola
Lady Caine
Mama Coca
Base
Basa
Barbs
Bazulco
Beam
Boy
Burese
Carnie
Candy C
Came
C-Dust
Cholly
Combol
Duct
Esnortiar
El Perico
Jelly
Mosquitos
Monster
Teenager
Tardust
Yesco
Yesca
Zambi

Amphetamines

Germany developed amphetamines in 1887. By the early 1900's amphetamines were being used for asthma and as energy supplements. World War II saw the development of amphetamine tablets which were given to soldiers on both sides to help them stay awake and alert. Following the war amphetamines became commonly used drugs for students and many professions which required the worker to stay awake or alert. Many cocaine users switched over because amphetamines gave them similar effects, but were cheap and readily available. Athletes also used amphetamines for the heightened energy, performance, and alertness it provided.

In the 1960's the FDA (Food and Drug Administration) restricted the use of amphetamines, making them controlled substances. Over the next several decades the use of amphetamines for medical purposes declined, as other medications were developed which have less side effects. There are still some formulations used for Attention Deficit Disorder (ADD), Attention Deficit with Hyperactivity Disorder (ADHD), and for Narcolepsy.

Amphetamines inhibit the re-uptake of Dopamine and Serotonin from the space between the neurons, causing an increased dopamine effect. They also cause increased norepinephrine in the brain and the blood, which is then converted into epinephrine (adrenaline). There is an additional indirect acetylcholine effect from amphetamines. Once again, therefore, we see the reason for the addiction potential of these drugs. Given in therapeutically appropriate doses (prescription doses), amphetamines tend to have very little adverse effects. They also have been shown to decrease hyperactivity and disruptive behaviors, as well as increasing focus and concentration. Given to individuals with ADD and ADHD they tend to have the opposite of what would be expected by giving someone a stimulant. Rather than stimulating activity, they increase focus, attention, and performance, minimizing impulsivity and hyperactivity.

When abused, amphetamines are generally taken in much higher doses than the prescription doses. These high doses often lead to rapid tolerance and dependence. Adverse effects from these high doses are potentially the same as other stimulants, as listed at the beginning of this chapter.

Unfortunately, amphetamines are still one of the products used for athletic "doping." Known effects of amphetamines include increased stamina, increased strength, increased endurance, increased acceleration, and decreased reaction time. Of course, using them at doses that provide these benefits are also doses that have high risk for addiction and the adverse effects of amphetamine use.

Methamphetamine

Methamphetamine (often called "meth"—not to be confused with methadone—which is an opiate) is related to amphetamines, and was developed in Japan in 1919. It was much more potent, easier to make, and soluble in water and therefore easily injectable. It was also used widely during World War II as a soldier enhancement project, on both sides of the war. After the war, it was also used as a stimulant, diet aid, antidepressant, and more. It was widely used and widely abused. In 1970, the US government made it illegal except by prescription. Drug gangs then began to be the primary producers until the Mexican drug cartels began massive production in the 1990's. Over the past 2 decades small labs have popped up in homes and small local labs increasing local regional

AMPHETAMINES

dextroamphetamine/ amphetamine:	Adderall Adderall XR
dextroamphetamine	Dexedrine ProCentra

AMPHETAMINE OVERDOSE

Cardiac arrhythmia
Confusion
Irritability
Hypertension
Muscle pain
Urinary retention
Tremors
Rapid breathing
Cardiogenic shock
Circulatory collapse
Hyperthermia
Renal failure
Psychosis
Seizures
Coma
Serotonin syndrome

AMPHETAMINE WITHDRAWAL

Fatigue
Irritability
Increased appetite
Abnormal dreams
Anxiety
Cravings
Sleep abnormalities
Movement disorders

STREET NAMES OF METHAMPHETAMINE [7]

Meth

Beanies
Brown
Chalk
Crank
Chicken feed
Cinnamon
Crink
Crypto
Fast
Getgo
Methlies quik
Mexican Crack
Pervitin
Redneck cocaine
Speed
Ticktick
Tweak
Wash
Yaba
Yellow powder

Crystal Meth

Batu
Blade
Cristy
Crystal
Crystal glass
Glass
Hot ice
Ice
Quartz

supplies. However, there is still a very large flow of methamphetamine up through the Rocky Mountain corridor from Mexico, coming across the border in a myriad of ways, such as dissolved in tequila. It is cheaper than cocaine, and has many of the same effects. Because of this, many cocaine users have transitioned to meth use instead.

Local meth labs have received much media attention, and with good reason. They are very dangerous, as the ingredients are highly toxic and explosive. Since they often pop up in kitchens, the risks associated with them are then transferred to anyone within the home, from the elderly to the infant. In attempts to try and curb the local production of methamphetamine, limitations have been imposed on the acquisition of various ingredients used to make methamphetamine, such as pseudo-ephedrine. Despite such restrictions, other processes are being developed to use different compounds.

Methamphetamine is available as a prescription, and if used for the proper indications, at the correct doses, it can be safe and effective. The brand name Desoxyn and the generic methamphetamine are both indicated for ADHD and for obesity. In either situation, the medication should be monitored very closely and prescribed with great care.

The current street forms of methamphetamine are much more potent and toxic than were the original formulations. The mechanism behind the action of methamphetamine is the frightening component. Like amphetamines, methamphetamine decreases the re-absorption of the dopamine from the nerve synapses. However, in addition to this, methamphetamine induces excess dopamine secretion from the afferent neuron. This dramatically increases the dopamine effect. Thus, we see the intensity of the motor responses and euphoria associated with dopamine release, and understand why it is so much more intense than many other drugs. Tragically, by inducing such extreme release of the dopamine, methamphetamine actually burns out the dopamine producing cells, and over time irreversibly damage the ability of the nerve cell to produce dopamine. Over time we may begin to see a Parkinson's Disease-like syndrome develop, which is caused by a lack of dopamine production.

The euphoria from methamphetamine is so high that users quickly become addicted. However, it is also short. A large amount of the methamphetamine remains in the system for several hours, and users have discovered that rapidly repeating the dose over and over will produce a recurrence of the high with much less of the drug being used. Many go on a "run," using it for days with very little food or sleep to maintain that high before they "crash." The intensity of the dopamine release is such that meth users' health can decline incredibly rapidly, as seen by the public education initiatives, depicting pictures of previously healthy individuals who are now emaciated and covered with self-inflicted sores.

Methamphetamine use has many severe and tragic side effects. Many of these are mentioned above in the list of effects. However, one of the very serious effects is the period of time known as "tweaking." This is the period of time when the drug level in the blood stream has dropped below the level at which it will make one "high." This period of time is potentially very dangerous, with hallucinations and psychosis to the point that the drug user self-mutilates, such as digging holes in their flesh because they are seeing, hearing, and feeling bugs burrowing under their skin. They can become violent and dangerous during this time.

Between the "runs," the "crashes," and the "tweaking," it is easy to see why a normal healthy individual can transform over a matter of only a few years into a scarred, sickly, emaciated individual who is spiraling rapidly towards death. The most important concept to understand here is that methamphetamine is one of the most addictive substances of abuse, and assuming one is immune to the addiction is literally playing with death, or at least such a tragic devastation to their health that they may never be the same.

Moreover, even if they are able to gain sobriety and abstinence from the drug, they may never again feel normal, as the brain remembers that intense high produced by the drug. If one survives methamphetamine use they are very likely to suffer from the many devastating physical symptoms from the damage to the dopamine system. A brief study of Parkinson's symptoms should be enough to convince anyone interested in trying methamphetamine to simply not do it. Sadly, no one ever begins such things expecting to experience such tragic outcomes. Most people who begin to use drugs assume that they are immune, and it will never happen to them. Tragically, drugs of any sort, but especially methamphetamine, are merciless masters.

METH EFFECTS

Short Term:

Agitation
Erratic behavior
Hallucinations
Skin picking
Convulsions
Overdose, death
Disordered sleep
Tachycardia
Hypertension
Hyperthermia
Nausea
Violence
Psychosis

Long Term:

Multiple organ failure
Skin destruction
Dental destruction
Lung disease
Nasal tissue destruction
Circulation destruction
Strokes
Heart attacks
Anorexia
Malnutrition
Confusion
Psychosis
Depression
Wasting syndrome
Dementia
Seizures
Liver failure
Kidney failure
Paranoia

METHAMPHETAMINE WITHDRAWAL [8]

"tweaking" – several hours to days:

Loss of sense of identity
Intense itching
Hallucinations, visual and auditory
Feeling of bugs crawling under skin
Psychosis
Violence, hostility
Self-mutilation

"crash" – several days:

Sleepy, listless, unresponsive

"hangover" – several days to weeks:

Deteriorated health
Dehydrated, malnourished
Physical and emotional exhaustion
Cravings

"withdrawal" – up to several months:

Depression
Loss of energy
Loss of pleasure
Severe cravings
Suicidality
Severe pain
Relapse, return to use

Phentermine

Phentermine is a stimulant that is used for weight loss. It is controlled and is listed as having a low to moderate risk of abuse potential. The medication is indicated for weight loss in obese persons. It has some typical effects for stimulants, primarily decreasing appetite. However, most people have to take it in the morning or it disrupts their sleep schedule. Because of the chance of addiction and abuse, this medicine should be used with caution, under a doctor's supervision.

Phentermine	Adipex-P
	Suprenza

APPENDIX H

Dissociative and Hallucinogenic Drugs

This class of drugs work on serotonin in the brain, as well as disrupting the glutamate activity on the NDMA receptors. This causes hallucinations, meaning seeing things, hearing things, and even feeling things that do not exist. Yet these hallucinations seem very real to the one experiencing these perceptions. They are, essentially, episodes of drug-induced psychosis. During these episodes, the user truly cannot perceive reality from psychosis.

There are short term effects from these drugs, which generally produce the effects for which these drugs are used. A "trip" refers to the experience one has after using these drugs. While the intent is to have a "good trip," any of these drugs can also produce a "bad trip." The results of use can vary with every use, depending on what is used, how much, and any factor around the person using, such as environment, mood, and more.

Effects of taking the drug generally begin anywhere from thirty to ninety minutes after use of the drug. The bad trips are unpredictable and can cause severe nightmares, terrors, anxiety, and feelings of impending doom and death. This may partly account for some of the terrible long-term consequences of using hallucinogens, which can lead to psychosis and personality disorders.

Long-term effects of hallucinogen use include two primary categories. The first is a persistent psychosis. The second is Hallucinogen Persisting Perception Disorder. "Long-term effects" does not mean that it requires use over long

DISSOCIATIVE DRUGS

LSD
Psilocybin
Peyote (mescaline)
PCP
Ketamine
Dextromethorphan
Marijuana

SHORT TERM EFFECTS OF HALLUCINOGENS [1]

- Hallucinations, including seeing, hearing, touching, or smelling things in a distorted way or perceiving things that do not exist
- Intensified feelings and sensory experiences (brighter colors, sharper sounds)
- Mixed senses ("seeing" sounds or "hearing" colors)
- Changes in sense or perception of time (time goes by slowly)

term. "Long-term effect" actually refers to the persistence of the effect of the drugs which may occur even after only a single use.

Tolerance develops rapidly with these drugs, and one develops a need to use more and more of the drug very quickly. However, after cessation of use, the tolerance also rapidly disappears. There are also rarely withdrawals symptoms with the cessation of use in this particular class of drugs.

These types of drugs produce various symptoms of mental and emotional detachment. Because of the out-of-body and other-worldly sensations they cause, they have often been interpreted as creating a "spiritual" experience. Historically these drugs have been used in religious ceremonies to create the feeling of having visions and other divine communications.

LONG-TERM EFFECTS OF HALLUCINOGENS

Persistent psychosis:

- Visual disturbances
- Disorganized thinking
- Paranoia
- Mood disturbances

HALLUCINOGEN PERSISTING PERCEPTION DISORDER (HPPD) [2]

- Hallucinations
- Other visual disturbances (such as seeing halos or trails attached to moving objects)
- Symptoms sometimes mistaken for neurological disorders (such as stroke or brain tumor)

STREET NAMES OF LSD

acid
blotter
doses
hits
microdots
sugar cubes
tabs
window panes

HALLUCINOGENS:

LSD (d-lysergic acid diethyl amide)

LSD is the popular name of a compound derived from a fungus that grows on rye. In its pure form it is odorless, tasteless, and colorless. It is generally used orally, but can be injected. During the 1940's it was isolated and marketed as a treatment for psychiatric disorders. Various uses were attempted during the 1950's, before it became popular in the 60's drug culture. Due to the severity of side effects with very little clinical benefit the drug became prohibited. The DEA has never found a legitimate medical use for LSD. In recent years medical research has again begun to see if there is any benefit in treatment of psychiatric illness. The onset of activity with LSD is 30-90 minutes, with an approximate twelve-hour duration. It most likely derives its effects by interrupting serotonin receptors, which are found throughout the body. Part of a syndrome common to LSD is "flashbacks," or sudden recurrence of the strange experiences which occurred during use of the drug. These may occur a day or even a year after the drug use. They may be so intense as to cause severe panic, anxiety, and paranoia, as well as having a severe negative impact on an individual's social and work environments.

The most common forms of LSD are tablets, capsules, gelatin squares, or tiny pieces of paper saturated with the drug. Whatever the form, LSD is known as likely the most potent reality and mood changing of drugs. Many consider as the standard against which to compare other hallucinogenic drugs. The drug was so popular in the 1960's and into the 1970's that references to it are still well understood, such as the reference made to it in Star Trek IV: The Voyage Home (1986), when Captain Kirk makes a reference to Spock, mistakenly explaining his strange behavior on "…too much LDS in the sixties," comically cross-referencing LSD use with the sometimes perceived "strange" behaviors of members of The Church of Jesus Christ of Latter-day Saints, though in reality there is no connection aside from a similar sounding acronym. [6, 7, 8, 9]

EFFECTS OF LSD [3]

- Increased blood pressure, heart rate, and body temperature
- Dizziness and sleeplessness
- Loss of appetite, dry mouth, and sweating
- Numbness, weakness, and tremors
- Impulsiveness and rapid emotional shifts that can range from fear to euphoria, with transitions so rapid that the user may seem to experience several emotions simultaneously

Psilocybin (4-phosphoryloxy-N,N-dimethy-Itryptamine)

Shrooms, or mushrooms, have long been a source for recreational and "religious" hallucinatory experiences. Psilocybin is the chemical responsible for these hallucinatory qualities. It is broken down into a chemical that acts on serotonin receptors. An article entitled "Groovy, Baby! Magic mushrooms & LSD Can Cure Depression—Study" actually does a good job of describing the effects of psilocybin.

> "A new study reveals the similarity between the way our brain works while sleeping, and when we're tripping on psychedelic drugs…
>
> "According to the scientists, taking psychedelic drugs is not only about rainbow-colored geometrical pictures popping up in the mind. Its effects on the brain not only cause changes in primitive areas of the brain linked to emotions and memory, but also tend to make people do less high-level thinking, and feel less self-conscious. All in all, brain activity becomes more disjointed and uncoordinated, immersing those experimenting with hallucinogenic drugs into a vivid, dreamlike state." [4]

This, of course, is not anything new to us. We have been aware of those dream-like hallucinatory effects of psilocybin for ages. Some people feel a dream-like world is preferable to real life.

STREET NAMES OF PSILOCYBIN

caps	hombrecitos
magic mushrooms	las mujercitas
mushrooms	little smoke
shrooms	Mexican mushrooms
cybin	musk
psilocyn	sacred mushrooms
god's flesh	silly putty
purple haze	simple simon
mushies	Mixed with MDMA
freedom caps	flower flipping
liberty caps	hippie flip
hippie stew	disco biscuits
boomers	

EFFECTS OF PSILOCYBIN [5]

- Feelings of relaxation (similar to effects of low doses of marijuana)
- Nervousness, paranoia, and panic reactions
- Introspective/ "spiritual experiences"

STREET NAMES OF PEYOTE

buttons
cactus
mesc
Devil's Root
dumpling cactus
Lophophora Williamsii
magic mushrooms
Mescal Buttons
Pellote
sacred mushrooms
Peyoti

PEYOTE SHORT TERM EFFECTS

altered perception
altered feeling
increased heart rate
increased blood pressure
increased body temperature
anorexia
insomnia
numbness
weakness
tremors

This dream-like state can be euphoric and wonderful, or terrible and horrifying. The state of the mind while being monitored is described as "disordered" or "disorganized." It is described as having a "mystical" experience. [10, 11, 12]

Peyote (Mescaline) Mescaline

Peyote (Mescaline)Mescaline is a hallucinogen derived from Peyote, a small thornless cactus native to Northern Mexico and the Southwestern United States. It has long been used for religious and medicinal purposes by the native populations of those areas. It is used orally, by chewing on the dried tops of the cactus, or by boiling it for tea.

In effect, it is very similar to LSD, though seemingly less potent. However, it can cause the same long-term effects, including Persistent Psychosis (PP) as well as Hallucinogen Persisting Perception Disorder (HPPD), even after just one use. The hallucinatory effects can persist for up to twelve hours. The "trips" can be pleasant and euphoric or terrifying. It is illegal in the United States, but is still used by native populations.

Mescaline works primarily by disrupting the neurotransmitter serotonin. Serotonin has a broad range of activity in the body, and much of the effect of mescaline can be understood by understanding what serotonin does. (See Appendix K). [13, 14, 15]

Dissociative Drugs

PCP (Phencyclidine)

During the 1950's PCP was developed to be used as an anesthetic. Unfortunately, it had such terrible side effects (confusion, delusions, irrational behavior) that it was discontinued in 1965. Street use began in the 1960's, but it was deemed too dangerous, and was mostly avoided. Use declined into the early 1990's, but has since began to increase slightly. PCP gives a person the illusion of being invincible, strong, and powerful, which seems to be the main appeal for ongoing use.

PCP is a white crystalline powder that can be used as capsules, tablets, powder, or liquid. It can be swallowed, snorted, or inhaled. When inhaled it is often applied to plant material that can burn, such as parsley, marijuana, mint, etc. Unlike the hallucinogens, PCP is addictive, inducing an ongoing pursuit of the drug.

If an extremely agitated, violent, and psychologically unstable person is brought into an emergency room it is not uncommon to screen for PCP, despite the fact that we do not often see PCP use. The drug has such a reputation for creating a severely aggressive and psychiatrically unstable patient that emergency personnel remember this drug. Many stories float around about the PCP user who is shot in a conflict but continues to attack despite being mortally wounded.

PCP binds to the NMDA/glutamate receptor. It also may have some effect on dopamine, nicotinic, and opiate receptors. [16, 17, 18]

Ketamine

After PCP was taken off the market as an anesthetic, Ketamine replaced it. Ketamine is structurally similar to PCP, but is much safer and more effective for anesthetic purposes. It has been used in battlefield injuries and in burn injuries, as well as in pediatric medicines wherein the patient does not tolerate other medications, and in veterinary medicine. Ketamine binds to the NMDA receptors and the opiate receptors

Unfortunately, Ketamine has become another abused drug due to its dissociative characteristics. It can be injected, eaten, or smoked, and is frequently added to marijuana. Due to its dissociative properties which can include confusion and amnesia, Ketamine has become a popular club drug, often used at "rave" parties, and also used as a date rape drug. It is odorless and tasteless and can be easily added to a drink. Unsuspecting partiers may be given a dose. It may cause them to be unable to speak or move, and can cause amnesia. This results in sexual assault with no recollection of the event.

Abuse of ketamine can cause out-of-body experiences, or a feeling of complete dissociation. These episodes are also known as "K-holes" or "near-death" experiences.

EFFECTS OF PCP

- delusions
- hallucinations
- paranoia
- confusion
- dissociation from reality
- anxiety
- depression
- suicidality
- memory loss
- disordered speech
- weight loss
- hypotension
- hypertension
- bradycardia
- tachycardia
- tachypnea
- hyperthermia
- nausea
- vomiting
- visual disturbances
- drooling
- loss of balance
- violence
- seizures
- coma
- accidental injury
- analgesia
- sense of strength
- sense of invulnerability
- rapid eye movements
- blank stare
- persistent speech problems

STREET NAMES FOR PCP

- Angel Dust
- Hog
- Ozone
- Rocket Fuel
- Shermans
- Wack
- Crystal
- Embalming Fluid
- PeaCe Pill
- Lovely
- Dust

WITH MARIJUANA

- Killer Joints
- Super Grass
- Fry
- Lovelies
- Wets
- Waters

EFFECTS OF KETAMINE

dissociation	violent behavior
addiction	depression
withdrawal	euphoria
lethargy	vomiting
delirium	nausea
sedation	numbness
chest pain	amnesia
hallucinations/ terrors	seizures
respiratory depression	coma
tachycardia	death
loss of coordination	bladder spasms
muscle rigidity	incontinence
	renal failure

BRAND NAMES FOR KETAMINE

Ketaset	Ketanest
Ketalar	Ketanest S
Ketalar SV	

STREET NAMES FOR KETAMINE

Special K	Super Acid
K	Green
Kit Kat	Special La Coke
Super C	Purple
Super Acid	Vitamin K
Cat Valium	bump
Jet	honey oil

SLANG FOR EXPERIENCES

k-land	God
K-hole	near death
baby food	

Ketamine is available through medical sources in the United States. However, Mexico is a major supplier of illicit ketamine used within the United States. [19, 20, 21, 22]

Dextromethorphan (DXM)

Found in many cough medicines, DXM is a chemical similar to morphine, which suppresses coughs during illness. It was developed as a safer alternative to codeine for cough suppression. At the prescribed dose, this is a very safe medication (though it should not be taken during pregnancy). However, abusers have discovered that at high doses it has some dissociative characteristics. It is commonly mixed with marijuana, ecstasy, and alcohol for the additive effects of the drugs. Alone or in combination it can create a feeling of being disconnected from the environment, as well as distorting one's emotions and changing one's perceptions. On rare occasions brain damage can occur from lack of oxygen to the brain.

There has been a dramatic increase in use since 2000, probably due to the club drug scene, and the availability and inexpensiveness of DXM compared to other illicit drugs. In 2008, one in ten teens admitted to abusing cough and cold medicines for the DXM effects, making it more commonly abused than cocaine, ecstasy, LSD, and meth. DXM is perceived by youth as being "safer" than other illicit drugs, partly because it is readily accessible over the counter in over a hundred cough and cold medicines.

Unfortunately, many parents have no idea that DXM is a problem, or even abusable. It is common in most homes, but bottles of cold medicines lying around do not seem as alarming as other drug paraphernalia. Most parents would

STREET NAMES FOR DXM

Dex	Skittles	Vitamin-D
DXM	Syrup	Vitamin-D
Robo	Triple-C	Tussin

not even consider a pre-teen abusing drugs, but even elementary age children are abusing cough and cold medicines. DXM can be obtained at very concentrated doses over the internet, making it more potent and much more dangerous. By the time kids get into college DXM is generally left behind for other drugs which are perceived to be more potent and more sophisticated. Combining DXM with other drugs is also quite common as a way to enhance the drug effects. [23, 24, 25]

HIGH DOSE DXM EFFECTS

- dissociative effects (similar to ketamine and PCP)
- distorted perceptions
- distorted emotions
- impaired motor function
- numbness
- nausea
- vomiting
- tachycardia
- arrhythmia
- slurred speech
- hypertension
- hypoxic brain injury
- hallucinations
- impaired vision
- sweating
- fever
- tachypnea
- memory loss
- coma
- rapid eye movements

APPENDIX I

BARBITURATES

BARBITURATES

Generic	Brand
amobarbital	Amytal
pentobarbital	Nembutal
secobarbital	Seconal
phenobarbital	
amobarbital and secobarbital	Tuinal
allobarbital	
aprobarbital	
alphenal	
brallobarbital	
barbital	

"9% of Americans will abuse a barbiturate at some time in their life. One in five children grow up in households where another member of the household abuses barbiturates or other drugs." [1]

Barbiturates were first developed in the 1860's, but not used for medical applications until the early 20th century. Barbiturates were discovered to have useful properties, including sedation, anesthesia, induction of anesthesia, and treating anxiety and insomnia. Short-acting barbiturates have been particularly useful for anesthesia, as they act quickly, and can be stopped with rapid recovery if there are complications.

Longer acting barbiturates, such as phenobarbital, have proven to be effective anticonvulsants. For this reason, phenobarbital is still sometimes used to keep people from having seizures during alcohol withdrawal, or benzodiazepine withdrawal. Phenobarbital is very slowly metabolized, and it takes about eighty hours for the body to remove half of the medication from the body (half-life). This is very useful after stopping long acting benzodiazepines, as their abrupt cessation may induce seizures.

By the 1950's, however, the risks of barbiturate use had become apparent, though they were still commonly used and popular into the 1970's. The risk of physical dependence and severe behavioral changes from using barbiturates moved this class of medicines to the sideline as treatments for anxiety and insomnia. Benzodiazepines became the drug of choice for treating these disorders.

The regular use of barbiturates rapidly leads to a tolerance, with rapid dose escalation. That, along with the mood-altering effects of the class make them potentially addictive. In addition to the addictive properties of barbiturates, sudden withdrawal can be life threatening.

When barbiturates are used, they have to be used very carefully. The difference between the dose that causes sedation and the dose that is lethal is very small. In controlled situations, with careful dosing, barbiturates, such as pentobarbital, are still used effectively and safely for sedation and anesthesia during medical procedures.

Barbiturate use, despite declining after the 1970s due to the dangerous nature of the class, seem to be on the rise again. On the street, they are used for the purpose of calming the less desirable effects of stimulant drugs. Barbiturates are also used to obtain a progressive state of disinhibition and intoxication, much like alcohol, but are much more likely to lead to coma and death. Because of this they are sometimes used in suicide attempts. Barbiturates are also used in lethal injections for capital punishment and for euthanasia.

Barbiturates work by binding to a GABA sub-receptor. By binding to the sub-receptor, they increase the GABA effect at the receptor. As previously explained, GABA is the primary inhibitory receptor in mammals, thus barbiturates disinhibit mammals relative to mood and decision making (thus the benzodiazepine-like and alcohol-like effects). Barbiturates also block a subtype of the glutamate receptor. Glutamate is the principle physiologic excitatory neurotransmitter in mammals. Thus, barbiturates inhibit the excitatory system in mammals, causing relaxation and sedation (alcohol also inhibits glutamate receptors, again explaining alcohol-like effects of barbiturates).

With this in mind it is important to understand the effects of combining alcohol with barbiturates, or benzodiazepines with barbiturates. In both cases the effect is additive. In addition, barbiturates enhance the effect of benzodiazepines, increasing the receptor sensitivity, and therefore making the dose of the benzodiazepine much more potent, and therefore much more dangerous than it would have normally been. In this way, they are not only addictive but compound the effects and the dangers of benzodiazepines.

STREET NAMES [2]

Amobarbital: Downers, blue heavens, blue velvet, blue devils

Pentobarbital: Nembies, yellow jackets, abbots, Mexican yellows

Phenobarbital: Purple hearts, goof balls

Secobarbital: Reds, red birds, red devils, lilly, F-40's, pinks, pink ladies, seggy

Tuinal: Rainbows, reds and blues, tooies, double trouble, gorilla pills, F-66s

OTHER STREET NAMES FOR BARBITURATES

Barbs	Stumblers
Tanks	Red Dolls
Downers	Tootsies
Sleepers	Rainbows

The dosing of barbiturates is very important to understand. Tolerance to barbiturates develops rapidly with frequent use, and those who abuse them quickly must escalate their dose to get the desired effect. Unfortunately, someone who has not used barbiturates in the past could easily die of an overdose when those already using barbiturates share what seems to them a dose that would only produce a minimal effect. The tolerance also rapidly dwindles. Therefore, an individual could be using very high doses of barbiturates, with a high tolerance, stop for a time, and then go back to use and overdose on the amount that previously only barely give them a mild drug effect.

In addition, children and older adults do not metabolize barbiturates nearly as rapidly as young and middle-aged adults. To complicate this further, many toxins in our bodies are broken down into substances called "metabolites," which may still have very active characteristics. Some barbiturates are broken down into metabolically active metabolites, that the body then has to further

DRUG EFFECTS

Altered consciousness
Impaired cognition
Impaired judgement
Impaired coordination
Anxiolytic
Sedation, drowsiness
Skeletal muscle relaxation
Dis-inhibition
Intoxication, similar to alcohol
Incoordination
Depressed breathing
Slurred speech
Sluggishness
Irritability
Anesthesia
Coma
Death
Physical dependence
Psychological dependence

WITHDRAWAL SYMPTOMS

Tremors
Anxiety
Agitation
Seizures
Insomnia
Hallucinations
Fever
Neonatal withdrawal

break down to detoxify. This, in combination with the variation of metabolic activity found with tolerance to the drug as well as changes related to age make barbiturates very dangerous drugs for the elderly population if not used under very close supervision.

Barbiturates cross the placenta, and mothers who use barbiturates during pregnancy can cause toxic effects to the fetus, and can deliver a barbiturate addicted infant. Barbiturates also pass into breast milk, and can therefore present all the risks of barbiturate use to a nursing baby.

Chronic use of barbiturates can also produce long-term effects. Mood changes, irritability, memory problems, and a lower level of life function are all potential results.

With all these factors, it is easy to see why barbiturates are used only in select situations now. Their narrow therapeutic window (the difference between effective and dangerous dosing) makes them a risky medication when there are other medications which are more effective, and safer. Benzodiazepines, despite their drawbacks, have been much safer, and in many cases more effective than the barbiturates. There are some alternatives for anxiety medications. These were discussed in the appendix regarding benzodiazepines.

APPENDIX J

Miscellaneous Compounds

The world of drug abuse is ever changing. Unfortunately, those who promote drug abuse, varied though their motives may be, continue to push the discovery of new drugs. There is always a demand for more potent highs, less expensive compounds, more addictive properties, etc. Once one is caught in an addiction the brain drives a person to want more, and to want it more intensely. Experimentation increases, from moving on to stronger drugs, to combining different drugs, to experimenting with more and more toxic compounds. There is little logic or reason behind the concept of experimentation in more dangerous and destruction behaviors. However, this concept of increasingly destructive behavior speaks volumes about the power of addiction.

This powerful chemically driven condition of addiction is ever leading the charge to the development of new drugs. Such development is often made to sound progressive, or appealing by labeling the drugs or the behaviors with appealing phrases. The drug culture of the 60's and 70's was labeled with such phrases as "the new morality," "sex, drugs, and rock and roll," and "make love, not war." Now we hear phrases such as "ecstasy," "designer drugs," "rave parties," etc. This exploration has led to many drugs which are quite popular, have no legal or medicinal use, and have varying properties that lead to them being less easily categorized than the drugs thus far described. the following drugs are examples of a few of the more common such drugs.

Androgenic Anabolic Steroids

The abuse of steroids is very concerning. These drugs are legitimately used for various medical conditions wherein the body no longer makes the appropriate steroids. However, when abused the steroids are taken in much larger amounts, either orally or injected. This is a concern because there are many serious health risks in doing so, but also because of the reasons for which they are taken.

Most drugs are abused because they cause a high or euphoria. Steroids, on the other hand, are used by people who want to improve their performance, size, or to look better. These desires are given preference over some very deadly long-term effects from the steroids because of the high doses.

BRANDS OF STEROIDS [1]

- Androsterone
- Oxandrin
- Dianabol
- Winstrol
- Deca-durabolin
- Equipoise

Androgenic means that these steroids cause masculine characteristics, such as increased body hair, deeper voice, and large muscle mass. This occurs because they are anabolic, which essentially

HEALTH EFFECTS OF STEROIDS [2]

Acne, oily skin
Edema
Headaches
Diarrhea
Stomach pain, upset
Hypertension
Liver damaged
Heart disease
Elevated cholesterol
Behavior changes
Mood swings
Fatigue
Restlessness
Poor appetite
Insomnia
Reduced sex drive
Steroid cravings
Depression, suicide

Women:

Excess body and face hair
baldness
changes in menstrual cycle
deep voice
enlarged clitoris

Men:

Infertility
Baldness
Atrophy of testicles
Enlarged breasts
Prostate cancer risk

means they induce growth. At normal physiologic doses (the normal amount produced by the testicles and ovaries) we see the differences between men and women in physical build and gender characteristics.

Despite the desired effects of steroid use, prolonged use actually shrinks the testicles and decreases testosterone production. This often leads to infertility in men. There are many other dangerous effects of using anabolic steroids at high doses, as noted in the list above. [3]

STREET NAMES FOR STEROIDS [4]

Arnolds	Stackers	Juice
Gym Candy	Weight trainers	Hype
Pumpers	Gear	Pumpers
Roids		

Bath Salts

Bath salts are a collection of synthetic "designer drugs" similar to cathinone, an amphetamine-like drug derived from the khat plant. These drugs hit the market labeled as bath salts to avoid detection by law enforcement. They are now being marketed under several other names, again to avoid detection. Many new chemicals are being developed that are also marketed as bath salts, though their chemical formulations may be different, with different effects. These chemicals are not related to the fragrant or therapeutic compounds previously intended to be added to bath water. The drug forms of bath salts are often labeled "not for human consumption," another ploy to evade scrutiny by legal regulatory agencies.

The word about these drugs rapidly spread through the drug-abusing community, marketed as if they were a benign aid for a comfortable bath. This was such a sudden intrusion of illicit drug use into an unsuspecting market that it took several years for states to pass legislation banning the use or sale of these drugs. Unfortunately, the damage was already done. Many were already addicted, and the revolutionary new way of taking drugs to market led to many other such attempts. Even now we are seeing the same chemicals passing around under other creative names, such as "plant food."

The most common stimulant in bath salts is a chemical called methylenedioxypyrovalerone (MDPV). It has effects very similar to cocaine, but can stimulate the dopamine release in the brain ten times more than cocaine. Because of this some have reported cravings after use to be as intense as those caused by methamphetamine use. These synthetic cathinones are also being used to substitute for or contaminate other drugs, such as spice (synthetic marijuana) and MDMA (ecstasy). [5, 6, 7, 8]

STREET NAMES OF BATH SALTS

ivory wave
purple wave
vanilla sky
bliss
bloom
cloud nine
lunar wave
white lightning
scarface
drone
meph
meow meow

SYNTHETIC CATHINONES

methylenedioxypyrovalerone (MDPV)
mephedrone
methedrone
pyrovalerone
butylone
naphyrone

SOME MARKETING NAMES

bath salts
plant food
jewelry cleaner
phone screen cleaner
cosmic blast

EFFECTS OF BATH SALTS

stimulant effects
euphoria
increased sociability
increased sex drive
agitation
paranoia
hallucinations/delusions
chest pain
increased pulse
increased blood pressure
suicidality
post-use agitation
psychosis
violent behavior
panic attacks
dehydration
muscle breakdown
death
seizures

Ecstasy, MDMA (3,4-methylenedioxy-methamphetamine)

Also known as "Molly", this drug has a combination of effects, partly a stimulant similar to amphetamine, partly a hallucinogen similar to mescaline. Ecstasy is commonly used at "raves" as a club drug. The popular effect of this drug is a feeling of increasing energy, along with a dramatic increase in empathetic feelings towards others. Users have an intense feeling of being able to understand others, and to be understood emotionally. This is likely due to MDMA causing a large release of serotonin in the brain, which influences mood, sleep, and appetite.

Serotonin also causes the release of oxytocin and vasopressin, two hormones that increase feelings of love, trust, sexual arousal, empathy, and emotional closeness. MDMA also induces increased effects of dopamine and norepinephrine. This combination results in increased stimulation and heightened sensations of energy. It is often used during concerts and dances to increase energy and endurance, as well as increasing emotional stimulation. The effects of the drug last anywhere from three to six hours. Doses are often repeated during all night raves.

The overstimulation of these three neurotransmitters then result in predictable deprivation syndromes, withdrawals, and cravings, due to depletion of those neurotransmitters. As is typical

STREET NAMES

ecstasy
molly (for "molecular")

Short-term effects of MDMA

increased heart rate
increased blood pressure
muscle tension
involuntary muscle clenching
nausea
blurred vision
faintness
chills
sweating
hyperthermia (overheated)
liver failure
kidney failure
heart failure
death

Long-term effects of MDMA

long-lasting confusion
depression
anxiety
sleep disorders
multi-organ damage

with most drugs, resultant effects of coming off the drug include anxiety, depression, and poor sleep. Some individuals suffer long-term confusion as well as problems with attention and memory.

Raves are extended parties, involving dancing and drug use. Because of the increased muscle tone and hyperthermia, dehydration is a very real risk at a rave. Also, because of the increased muscle tone they experience involuntary teeth clenching. Participants often have pacifiers in their mouth to help protect their teeth from being damaged during their episodes of drug intoxication.

More and more ecstasy is being adulterated with other drugs as additives. These include ephedrine, dextromethorphan, ketamine, caffeine, cocaine, methamphetamine, and cathinones. Such combinations make the MDMA even more toxic and dangerous. It is also being used with sildenafil (Viagra), for improved sexual function to go along with the increased sexual drive, dramatically increasing the risks of sexually transmitted diseases. [9, 10, 11]

GHB (Gamma Hydroxybutyrate)

This drug is particularly well known as a "date rape" drug. It is also used in raves, and is often added to alcoholic beverages, intentionally or covertly. It is odorless, tasteless, and colorless, and has often been added to unsuspecting persons' drinks, rendering them sedated and sometimes incapacitated, vulnerable to sexual assault. It may also cause amnesia, leaving them with no memory of being assaulted. Additionally, the drug itself can cause euphoria, increase sex drive, and make one feel tranquil, all adding to the risk of sexual victimization.

GHB is bought off the streets, or on the internet. It comes as a clear liquid, or a white powder. As with other drugs it is often adulterated with contaminants, including alcohol and other drugs, making it more dangerous, and more unpredictable. Unfortunately, overdoses are not unusual, as the dosing is not well understood by many who use it, and varies greatly depending on how it is made. It has many of the typical long-term effects of other drugs, including insomnia, anxiety, and permanent organ damage.

This drug, though very dangerous, is often used voluntarily by party-goers. It is not unusual for body builders to use it, as it has an anabolic effect on muscle, similar to steroids used in body-building. The effects of the drug are such that the federal registration for this drug lists it as a schedule I, meaning there is no approved medicinal purpose for GHB. In other words, the dangers of the drug far outweigh any beneficial effects from the drug.

STREET NAMES OF GHB

Liquid X	G	Great hormones at bedtime	GBH
Liquid ecstasy	Vita-G	Great hormones	Soap
Liquid E	G-juice	Somatomax	Easy lay
Georgia home boy	Liquid G	Bedtime scoop	Salty water
Oop	Fantasy	Gook	G-Riffick
Gamma-oh	Scoop	Gamma-10	Cherry Meth
Grievous bodily harm	Water	Energy drink	Organic Quaalude
Mills	Everclear		Jib

EFFECTS OF GHB

Central nervous system depression	Sweating	Vomiting	Clumsiness
Depressed breathing	Loss of consciousness	Aspiration	Amnesia
Euphoria	Nausea	Exhaustion	Seizures
Increased sex drive	Hallucinations	Sluggishness	Coma
Tranquility	Headaches	Confusion	Death

There is one formulation of a GHB salt derivative that was approved for severe sleep disorders with narcolepsy, called Zyrem. It is rigidly controlled, and access to the drug is restricted by special enrollment programs. [12, 13, 14]

Khat

Khat is another naturally occurring chemical from the shrub Catha edulis that is found in East Africa and the Arabian Peninsula. It is a stimulant, and acts similarly to methamphetamine or cocaine, though it is not as potent. It triggers norepinephrine release, and increases dopamine levels in the brain. The primary active chemical in it is the stimulant cathinone. Because of this it is illegal by federal regulations.

A large concern regarding khat is that chewing it is an accepted part of the culture of many countries. As those people immigrate to the United States, khat use is becoming more common, and the drug is becoming more available.

The fresh leaves are chewed (similar to chewing tobacco). If a fresh supply cannot be obtained then dried leaves are made into a paste and chewed, or the leaves are smoked or made into a tea. [15, 16, 17, 18]

EFFECTS OF KHAT

typical stimulant effects	increased alertness	increased heart rate	reduces fatigue
euphoria	increased arousal	increased blood pressure	reduces appetite

Withdral

depression	irritability	loss of appetite	insomnia

Long-term effects

tooth decay	esophageal cancer	worsening psychiatric disorders	anorexia
constipation	heart disease	liver damage	insomnia
stomach cancer	mood disorders		

STREET NAMES FOR KHAT

Qat	Miraa	African salad	Somali tea
Kat	Quadkaa	Bushman's tea	Tohai
Chat	Abyssinian tea	Oat	Tschat
Gat			

Krokodil

Krokodil is the street name for a codeine derivate being "cooked" in homes and labs as a drug of abuse. The name reportedly comes from the reptilian-like gangrene scale and scars in the body tissues after using the drug. It may also come from a parent compound called chlorocodide, developed during the cooking of codeine to derive desomoprhine, the opiate responsible for the euphoria of krokodil.

It has primarily been used in Russia, but there have been documented cases now in the United States. Russian use escalated dramatically from rare to astounding levels from 2005 to 2011. A national ban on over-the-counter sales of codeine in 2012 caused a plummet in the availability of krokodil, but codeine has again now become readily available on the black market.

Codeine is used to derive a highly potent and euphoric pain medicine called desomorphine. Desomorphine was originally developed in 1932 as a pain medicine, but was banned in 1936 in the United States because it was so highly addictive.

The compound is made using various toxic substances. These are generally not removed completely during the cooking process, and the compound sold as krokodil tends to be highly toxic. However, it produces such an intense "high" along with having a short duration of effect (about two hours) that there is an immediate return demand for the drug.

This is an incredibly unfortunate circumstance, as the toxic nature of this substance rapidly leads to tissue destruction. Injecting the drug into the veins destroys vessels and surrounding tissues, resulting in necrotic tissue, gangrene, loss of limbs, liver and kidney failure, brain damage, brain infections, and more. Attempts to inject the drug that miss the vein result in immediate tissue destruction, abscesses, loss of large portions of flesh or bone, and eventually the loss of limbs, and death. Because of this it has been dubbed the "zombie drug." It is difficult to express the horrible severity of the destruction caused by krokodil. Any curious party can quickly and easily find pictures of crippled victims on the internet, with huge portions of limbs and tissue missing, bones bare of flesh, rotting tissue literally falling from their bodies.

The intensity of the high along with the incredibly toxic nature of the drug make this an extremely dangerous substance to abuse, and a very difficult addiction to treat. The expected life span of an individual who begins using krokodil is two to three years. [19, 20]

STREET NAMES FOR DESOMORPHINE [19]

krokodil
Russian Magic
flesh-eating drug
Zombie drug
Cheornaya (in Russia)
Himiya (in Ukraine)

HEALTH HAZARDS OF KROKODIL [19]

blood vessel damage
open ulcers, gangrene, phlebitis
skin and soft tissue infections
skin grafts/surgery
limb amputations
pneumonia
blood poisoning
meningitis
rotting gums, tooth loss
blood borne virus transmission (HIV, Hepatitis C)
bone infections (osteomyelitis)
speech and motor skill impairment
memory loss and impaired concentration
liver and kidney damage
overdose
death

Rohypnol (flunitrazepam)

Rohypnol is actually a benzodiazepine called flunitrazepam. It is not available for prescription use in the United States. However, it is another commonly used drug at raves and parties. Rohypnol's effects are very similar to valium, but up to ten times as powerful in the sedative effects. It has been used for several reasons. Rohypnol has been popular in decreasing some of the negative effects of stimulants, particularly in decreasing the depression caused by methamphetamine and cocaine. It is also popular to enhance the effects of heroin. Rohypnol is also another drug used for "date rape," as it can cause sedation, relaxation, and amnesia of events while the drug is in the system. The manufacturer changed the formulation into a capsule with blue dye in it so it would be detectable if placed in a clear liquid. However, darker liquids will still hide it, and there are generic forms of flunitrazepam that do not have any coloring in them.

Rohypnol is still used legally in many countries, including Mexico and Europe, so it is not surprising that there is illicit access to this drug in the United States. As with other benzodiazepines, it is often combined with alcohol, which amplifies the effects of both, particularly the sedation and respiratory depression.[21, 22, 23]

STREET NAMES FOR ROHYPNOL

Forget-me pill	Roche	Ropies	Rope	Rophy
Mexican Valium	Roofies	Ruffels	Rophies	Rib
R2	Roopies	Roofinal		Roach-2

EFFECTS OF ROHYPNOL

Incapacitation	Loss of muscle control	Drowsiness	Decreased anxiety	Tolerance
Insomnia	Confusion	Sedation	Anti-convulsant	Dependence

LONG-TERM USE EFFECTS

Anxiety

Insomnia *See appendix on Benzodiazepines for class effects.*

Salvia (Salvia divinorum)

STREET NAMES FOR SALVIA

Shepherdess's herb	Magic mint
Diviner's sage	Sally-D
Seer's sage	Sage of the Seers
Maria pastora	Lady Salvia
	Purple sticky
	Sister Salvia

Salvia is an herb native to Mexico that has been used for centuries in religious rites amongst certain native populations. As a drug of abuse, it is relatively new on the scene of street drugs. Though it is generally considered a hallucinogen, it's function and effects are actually somewhat different than the other hallucinogens we have discussed. Whereas most of those work by triggering serotonin receptors, Salvia actually works on an opiate receptor, but a different receptor than the other opiates which are used for pain, or to get euphoria. Salvia actually works on an opiate receptor that depletes dopamine in the brain, resulting in hallucinations and dysphoric feelings.

The sudden popularity of Salvia may be due to internet posting of videos of people using Salvia. It is not a popular party drug or club drug, and the appeal seems to be mostly recording the "trips" and posting them on the internet. Thus far it does not appear to be a popular drug for repeated use, yet its use has escalated among teens over the past few years.

There is still limited information on the long-term effects of Salvia. Some consider it to be more psychoactive than LSD and cocaine, and different. Salvia seems to cause a dissociation of sensory perception, disconnecting some sensory, and connecting other sensory to systems that do not have the ability to perceive sensation. One example was an individual reporting that they could see with their skin. This drug is new enough that it is not yet been listed as illegal on a federal level, though some states have outlawed it. It is still for sale in some states in places such as gas stations and smoke shops. [25, 26, 27]

EFFECTS OF SALVIA [24]

hallucinations
sensory disconnect
mood changes
depression
anxiety
abnormal body sensations
emotional swings
psychosis
loss of coordination
slurred speech
dizziness
slurred speech
giggling, laughter
memory loss

Long-term Effects

still unknown
possible memory loss
possible learning impairment

Spice, K2, Synthetic Marijuana

Spice is a name given to a group of designer drugs that consist mostly of cannabinoids (marijuana is one type of cannabinoid). Spice has been skillfully marketed as an herbal, natural, safe substitute for marijuana. Spice, or variations of it, are actually plant materials packaged and sold as incense that can be smoked, which is actually plant material that is sprayed with chemicals which are various cannabinoids (chemicals similar to marijuana). As a rule, they produce similar effects to marijuana, though some of them are more potent. Because the chemicals are slightly different, they often do not test positive on regular drug screens which test for marijuana.

This group of compounds have been marketed under various names, again to disguise them from authorities. Since the active compounds are so similar to marijuana they have been classified as Schedule I substances, meaning they have no medicinal value, and are not approved for medical purposes. This, of course, slides into the ongoing debates surrounding the legalization of marijuana. For several years the compounds were sold at gas stations and in smoke shops, until studies showed that the active components were related to marijuana.

EFFECTS OF SPICE

Similar effects to marijuana
elevated mood
altered perception
relaxation
anxiety
hallucinations
paranoia
vomiting
agitation
confusion
panic attacks
giddiness
increased heart rate
increased blood pressure
heart attacks

Long-term effects:

unclear, too new.

STREET/TRADE NAMES FOR SPICE

Synthetic marijuana	Bliss	Solar Flare	The Moon	Ono Budz
K2	Bombay Blue	Pep Spice	G-Force	Panama Red Ball
K2 Blond	Genie	Fire n' Ice	Blueberry Haze	Puff
K2 Standard	Zohai	Zombie World	Dank	Sativah Herbal
fake weed	Zoh	Bad-to-the-Bone	Demon Passion	Smoke
Yucatan fire	Blaze	Blaze	Smoke	Skunk
Skunk	Red X Dawn	Dark Night	Hawaiian Hybrid	Ultra Chronic
Moon rocks	Spice Gold, Spice	Earthquake	Magma	Voodoo Spice
Black Mamba	Diamond	Berry Blend	Ninja	Aroma

Unfortunately, Spice and related products are very popular among high school students, second only to marijuana in illicit drug use. Many of the youth are under the impression that Spice is safer than other drugs because it has been marketed as "natural." It has also been labeled "not for human consumption," which helped it evade the attention of legal regulations for a time. Spice is generally smoked, but some people make it into a tea. [28, 29, 30]

APPENDIX K

NEUROTRANSMITTERS—A QUICK REFERENCE

This appendix is more technical in nature, and is not intended as a read-through appendix. Understanding neurotransmitters is necessary to understanding the effects of drugs on the body. However, the intent of this appendix is to be an easy reference, and can be used as a reference to understand the function of a particular neurotransmitter.

As previously discussed, a neurotransmitter is simply a chemical that is released at the end of one neuron (the basic cell type in the nervous system that conduct signals through our body), travels across the nerve synapse (the space between neurons), and triggers a signal or response in the next nerve. This response could be to excite the nerve, calm the nerve, or induce further signal transfer. Many neurotransmitters are involved in common addictions. We will discuss a few of the more common of these, what they do, and how they contribute to the addictive process.

The University of Utah has a very informative interactive website that helps understand the roles and effects of neurotransmitters on the brain:

http://learn.genetics.utah.edu/content/addiction/drugs/mouse.html

There are many more links at the University of Utah genetics website.

Below is a list of some of the neurotransmitters that are of more importance in our discussion of addiction, followed by a brief description of what they do, and why they are involved in addiction.

1. Acetylcholine
2. Adenosine
3. Aspartate
4. Dopamine
5. Epinephrine and Norepinephrine
6. GABA (gamma-aminobutryic acid)
7. Glutamate
8. Histamine
9. NMDA (N-methyl-D-aspartate) receptor
10. Opioid peptides
11. Serotonin

Acetylcholine

Acetylcholine is involved within the brain (central nervous system) as well as in the nerves outside the brain (peripheral nervous system). There are several types of receptors, and a variety of effects which acetylcholine has upon the body. For example, it may cause increased attention and focus. It may cause increased muscle contractions in our skeletal muscle, while calming the contractions of the heart muscle. Many medications and drugs target the acetylcholine receptors. This is a very useful neurotransmitter to understand.

One specific area important in addiction is understanding there are different types of receptors upon which acetylcholine acts. One of these is the nicotinic receptor. As can be guessed, nicotine is one of the compounds that affects these receptors, and can mimic acetylcholine. Caffeine can also trigger the release of acetylcholine, which contributes to the stimulant effects of caffeine.

Several diseases involve nicotine receptors. Myasthenia Gravis is a disorder of the Acetylcholine receptors, caused by the body producing antibodies that attack the receptors (auto-antibodies). Alzheimer's Disease is helped by the administration of drugs that affect the acetylcholine system, by increasing attention and sensory perception in those individuals.

Adenosine

Adenosine works upon several receptor sub-types. Adenosine affects many tissues, including heart and lungs. It also acts in the brain, as an **inhibitory neurotransmitter**. When our bodies are worn down and fatigued and we begin to deplete our resources, the release of adenosine puts a check on our activities, making us feel tired and sleepy. Such a natural braking system is critical for our bodies to rest, regenerate, and restore their normal function.

Caffeine's stimulant effects in the brain are primarily caused by binding to and blocking the adenosine receptor. Once that receptor is bound, adenosine cannot bind to it, causing inhibition of the inhibition. In other words, caffeine thwarts the body's safety valve. A short burst of such inhibition can be recovered from quickly. However, chronic inhibition of the bodies maintenance program is like refusing to do maintenance on a car or a building as it ages.

There are many other effects of adenosine in the body. It helps control energy transfer. It also influences sleep and wake cycles. It has many effects on the heart and circulatory tissues.

Aspartate

Aspartate is a form of the amino acid aspartic acid, first discovered in asparagus. It can act as a neurotransmitter by stimulating NMDA receptors. The NMDA receptor is also one of the targets of glutamate. Aspartate's action is very similar to glutamate, but not as potent.

Dopamine

Dopamine is perhaps the most important neurotransmitter in the disease process of addiction. Virtually every type of reward system in the brain involves dopamine. Not only does dopamine act as the primary neurotransmitter for reward systems, it also affects motor function and the release of various hormones. Any behavior that is important to the body causes dopamine release, such as eating, sexual behaviors, etc. Other behaviors can also cause dopamine release, such as shopping, gambling, or extreme sports. Many drugs cause dopamine release, such as stimulants, cocaine, amphetamine, opiates, etc.

The release of dopamine is so powerful in making us feel good that it reinforces whatever behavior caused the release. This is important in reinforcing activities that are essential to life, such as eating to avoid starvation, or sex which is essential to carry on our race. However, it can also be very destructive if the dopamine release becomes our primary motivation.

Many diseases are related to problems with the dopamine system, aside from addiction. Parkinson's disease results from the depletion of dopamine. This happens when dopamine releasing neurons are damaged in the brain. We have seen this disease induced by drug users who have used "contaminated" drugs, where the dopamine releasing cells are damaged and the develop a "Parkinson's-like" syndrome. We have also seen that many of the popular drugs can damage the neurons which release dopamine, and thus we would expect to see Parkinson's-like syndromes developing from certain types of drug abuse, even though they are not considered contaminated with other compounds.

Dopamine has many effects outside of the brain, in regulation of other organ functions. These systems are independent of each other, as dopamine does not cross through the blood-brain barrier. Dopamine in the blood will not affect the dopamine receptors in the brain. However, dopamine does affect the immune system, the kidneys, the pancreas, pain conditions, and many more organs and conditions.

On one occasion, I spoke to a group of youth about addiction, and explained the role of dopamine in addiction. Afterwards a man who had recently been diagnosed with Parkinson's Disease came up and talked to me. He told me that my explanations of dopamine helped him understand why he was suffering from many of the symptoms of his Parkinson's Disease. Whereas before he had been afraid of taking the medication he had been prescribed (a dopamine replacement), he now understood why taking the medicine would help him feel and function better. Thus, we can understand that dopamine is not only a feel-good neurotransmitter, but it is vital to our body's function.

Epinephrine (adrenaline) and Norepinephrine (noradrenaline)

These two chemicals are very similar in structure and activity. They can act as either hormones or neurotransmitters. Norepinephrine is synthesized from dopamine. These chemicals cause stimulation of the nervous system, including increased alertness, increased strength, and faster response times. They increase heart rate and blood pressure, dilate airways, improve visual perception, and all those things we associate with the "fight-or-flight" response. Memory of events can be enhanced, as well as overall performance. This response plays some role in addictions, but we primarily see it in individuals who are intentionally engaging in high risk behaviors. Such individuals have been referred to as "adrenaline junkies."

Epinephrine is frequently used medically, to treat allergic reactions, anaphylactic reactions, asthma and breathing conditions, and to resuscitate the heart if someone's heart stops suddenly. These chemicals are very useful medically, but do seem to have some connection to addiction behaviors.

Norepinephrine is very similar to dopamine in structure. It is responsible for focus and concentration. It also affects the rate of contractions in the heart. Consistent with the fight-or-flight response, it also triggers release of glucose and increased blood flow to skeletal muscle.

GABA (gamma-Aminobutyric acid)

In mammals, GABA is the primary **inhibitory neurotransmitter**. Many drugs act upon the GABA receptors. Therefore, the chemicals or drugs that bind to GABA receptors have an inhibitory effect. Examples include alcohol, barbiturates, benzodiazepines, carisoprodol, methaqualone, inhaled anesthetics, and more. In essence, when someone uses a chemical that can activate a GABA receptor, they slow the activity of the neuron attached to that receptor. Thus, effects of these drugs include relaxation, decreased anxiety, and anti-convulsant effects. Sometimes they also produce amnesia. On the other hand, chemicals that block the GABA receptors can lead to overexcitement of the nerves.

Glutamate

Glutamate is a salt derivative of Glutamic Acid, a non-essential amino acid. The salt derivative is best known by the product marketed for flavoring and tenderizing foods, monosodium glutamate (MSG). Glutamate was named after being extracted from wheat gluten.

Glutamate is involved in functions such as learning and memory. It is an **excitatory neurotransmitter**, meaning it activates, or excites, the next neuron. The target of Glutamate is the *N*-methyl-D-aspartate receptor (NMDA). When Glutamate activates the NMDA receptor it helps trigger learning, and establish memories within the brain. As one of the most abundant neurotransmitters, Glutamate is involved in many disease processes, such as Lou Gehrig's Disease, phenylketonuria, autism, Alzheimer's Disease, and mental retardation. Glutamate can be released in excess, or not reabsorbed by transporters which remove it from the synapse. Either situation can cause toxicity, which can lead to cell death.

Several chemicals act on the Glutamate receptors (NMDA receptor). Ketamine, dextromethorphan, and PCP (phencyclidine) can all cause a feeling of dissociation and can cause hallucinations. Alcohol reduces the effectiveness of Glutamate on the NMDA receptor, thus being at least partially responsible for memory loss that may occur during intoxication. Alcohol's suppression of this excitatory neurotransmitter is one of the things that makes alcohol a depressant, and sedative hypnotic.

Histamine

Histamines have many physiologic effects in addition to the neurotransmitter effects. They can cause relaxation of the airways, dilation of blood vessels, and all the typical allergy symptoms, such as itching, nausea, sedation, and more. Additionally, histamine receptors can alter the release of neurotransmitters, such as acetylcholine, norepinephrine, and serotonin. Histamine affects sleep, sexual function, stomach acid release, immune system function, allergies, breast milk production, and more. Therefore, any drug that affects histamine receptors can have very far reaching effects.

NMDA (N-methyl-D-aspartate) Receptor

NMDA is a receptor, not a neurotransmitter. However, it deserves special mention here due to the effects derived upon a person by activation of this receptor. It is primarily activated by glutamate, which was discussed previously. Dissociative drugs cause most of their effects by disrupting the effects of glutamate at the NMDA receptors. Activation of the NMDA receptors impact learning, memory, perception, emotion, and how one perceives pain. Short term and long-term effects of disrupting this particular receptor can be devastating.

Opioid Peptides

Opioid peptides are the body's own natural amino acid chains that trigger our brain's opiate receptors. We commonly hear about endorphins, enkephalins, dynorphins, nociceptin, etc. These are the chemicals that trigger our opiate receptors in a normal way. Our body needs these to help us when we experience stress or pain. These chemicals also help us with emotion, developing attachments, and being motivated to do things. Opioid peptides are essential to our function, our comfort, our relationships, and our life-sustaining behaviors. They function by inducing the release of dopamine, the "feel-good" drug which our body naturally makes to reinforce behaviors or events.

Opioid peptides are found in many places. Many foods contain opiate peptides, though they generally have little effect as they are broken down before crossing the blood-brain barrier. However, plant derived opiates in high concentrations were found millennia ago. These do have very useful effects in controlling severe pain, beyond the capacity of our own body to control certain types of pain. While beneficial in some ways, opiates can also be very destructive.

Serotonin

Serotonin is a neurotransmitter that is primarily involved in the gut. However, it does have significant impact on mood. It modulates memory, anxiety, depression, appetite, aggression, dopamine release, heart function, nausea, movement of food through the gut, appetite, aging, organ development, learning, memory, etc.

Many of the psychedelic drugs release serotonin, such as LSD and psilocin. MDMA (commonly known as ecstasy) causes increased serotonin release, which partially explains the sudden intense feelings of sympathy and intimacy of MDMA use. The antidepressants including monoamine oxidase inhibitors (MAOIs), tricyclics (TCAs), and selective serotonin reuptake inhibitors (SSRIs) and selective norepinephrine serotonin reuptake inhibitors (SNRI's) all effect serotonin levels.

High levels of serotonin can cause a condition known as serotonin syndrome. This is a very dangerous condition. It can lead to death if too much serotonin is released, or active in the body.

Appendix References

Research sources:

1. http://www.drugabuse.gov/drugs-abuse/commonly-abused-drugs/commonly-abused-drugs-chart
2. http://www.drugabuse.gov/drugs-abuse/commonly-abused-drugs/commonly-abused-prescription-drugs-chart
3. http://www.justice.gov/dea/druginfo/factsheets.shtml
4. http://www.getsmartaboutdrugs.com
5. www.drugfreeworld.org
6. http://www.drugabuse.gov

Introduction – Drugs of Addiction, Introduction

1. Extent of illicit drug use and dependence, and their contribution to the global burden of disease, Louisa Deneghardt, Wayne Hall, www.thelancet.com, p 55.

Appendix B – Tobacco/Nicotine

1. http://www.lung.org/stop-smoking/about-smoking/facts-figures/general-smoking-facts.html
2. http://bjp.rcpsych.org/content/154/6/797.short, http://www.sciencedirect.com/science/article/pii/S0006322300010945
3. http://www.webmd.com/smoking-cessation/understanding-nicotine-withdrawal-symptoms

Appendix C – Cannabinoids

1. http://www.drugabuse.gov/publications/drugfacts/high-school-youth-trends
2. http://casapalmera.com/nicknames-street-names-and-slang-for-marijuana/
3. http://casapalmera.com/nicknames-street-names-and-slang-for-marijuana/
4. http://casapalmera.com/nicknames-street-names-and-slang-for-marijuana/
5. http://alcoholism.about.com/od/pot/a/Marijuana-Withdrawal-Symptoms.htm
6. http://www.drugabuse.gov/publications/drugfacts/marijuana

Appendix D – Opiates and Opioids

1. http://www.emedicinehealth.com/barbiturate_abutse/topic-guide.htm
2. http://www.drugabuse.gov/drugs-abuse/commonly-abused-drugs-charts/commonly-abused-prescription-drugs-chart
3. http://www.opiaterehabtreatment.com/street-names-opiates
4. http://www.nlm.nih.gov/medlineplus/ency/article/000949.htm

Appendix E – Benzodiazepines

1. http://www.intheknowzone.com/substance-abuse-topics/sedatives-tranquilizers-a-analgesics/street-names.html
2. http://www.oceantwp.org/content/5927/80/289/317/905.aspx
3. http://www.deadiversion.usdoj.gov/drug_chem_info/benzo.pdf

Appendix F- Sedative Hypnotics and Sleepers

1. The Effect of Melatonin, Magnesium and Zinc on Primary Insomnia in Long-Term Care Facility Residents in Italy: A Double-Blind, Placebo-Controlled Clinical Trial, Rondanelli, January 2011, Journal of the American Geriatrics Society, Volume 59, Issue 1, pp. 82-90.

Appendix G – Stimulants

1. http://www.drugfreeworld.org/drugfacts/prescription/stimulants.html
2. http://stimulants.com/what-are-stimulants/common-stimulants-slang-names/
3. http://stimulants.com/types-of-stimulants/street-names-for-stimulants/
4. http://www.npr.org/blogs/thesalt/2013/01/22/170002123/energy-drinks-blamed-for-boom-in-emergency-room-visits
5. http://alcoholism.about.com/od/coke/a/Common-Street-Names-For-Cocaine.htm
6. http://www.drugabuse.gov/publications/research-reports/cocaine-abuse-addiction/what-treatments-are-effective-cocaine-abusers
7. http://www.drugfreeworld.org/drugfacts/crystalmeth/what-does-methamphetamine-look-like.html#streetnames
8. http://www.drugfreeworld.org/drugfacts/crystalmeth/the-stages-of-the-meth-experience.html

Appendix H – Dissociative and Hallucinogenic Drugs

1. http://www.drugabuse.gov/publications/research-reports/hallucinogens-dissociative-drugs/where-can-i-get-more-scientific-information-hallucinogens-diss
2. http://www.drugabuse.gov/publications/research-reports/hallucinogens-dissociative-drugs/where-can-i-get-more-scientific-information-hallucinogens-diss
3. http://www.drugabuse.gov/publications/research-reports/hallucinogens-dissociative-drugs/where-can-i-get-more-scientific-information-hallucinogens-diss
4. http://rt.com/news/170248-science-magic-mushrooms-brain/
5. http://www.drugabuse.gov/publications/research-reports/hallucinogens-dissociative-drugs/where-can-i-get-more-scientific-information-hallucinogens-diss
6. http://www.drugabuse.gov/publications/research-reports/hallucinogens-dissociative-drugs/what-are-dissociative-drugs
7. http://www.drugfreeworld.org/drugfacts/lsd.html
8. http://en.wikipedia.org/wiki/Lysergic_acid_diethylamide
9. http://www.drugabuse.gov/publications/drugfacts/hallucinogens-lsd-peyote-psilocybin-pcp
10. www.drugfree.org/drug-guide/mushrooms/
11. http://www.justice.gov/archive/ndic/pubs6/6038/
12. http://www.drugabuse.gov/publications/research-reports/hallucinogens-dissociative-drugs/what-are-facts-about-dissociative-drugs
13. http://www.drugfree.org/drug-guide/peyote/
14. http://www.drugabuse.gov/publications/drugfacts/hallucinogens-lsd-peyote-psilocybin-pcp
15. http://www.webmd.com/vitamins-supplements/ingredientmono-473-PEYOTE.aspx?activeIngredientId=473&activeIngredientName=PEYOTE
16. http://www.drugabuse.gov/publications/drugfacts/hallucinogens-lsd-peyote-psilocybin-pcp
17. http://www.deadiversion.usdoj.gov/drug_chem_info/pcp.pdf
18. http://www.drugs.com/illicit/pcp.html
19. http://www.drugs.com/illicit/ketamine.html
20. http://www.drugfreeworld.org/drugfacts/prescription/ketamine.html
21. http://www.deadiversion.usdoj.gov/drug_chem_info/ketamine.pdf
22. http://alcoholism.about.com/od/lsd/a/Basic-Facts-About-Ketamine.htm
23. http://teens.drugabuse.gov/drug-facts/dextromethorphan-dxm-and-cold-medicine
24. http://www.eaglevillehospital.org/PDFs/DXM.pdf
25. http://www.webmd.com/parenting/teen-abuse-cough-medicine-9/teens-and-dxm-drug-abuse

Appendix I – Barbiturates

1. www.emedicinehealth.com/barbiturate_abuse/article_em.htm
2. www.emedicinehealth.com/barbiturate_abuse/article_em.htm

Appendix J – Miscellaneous Compounds

1. http://teens.drugabuse.gov/drug-facts/anabolic-steroids

1. http://www.drugabuse.gov/drugs-abuse/commonly-abused-drugs/health-e ects#steroids

2. http://www.drugabuse.gov/publications/research-reports/anabolic-steroid-abuse/letter-director

3. http://www.deadiversion.usdoj.gov/drug_chem_info/anabolic.pdf

4. http://www.webmd.com/mental-health/addiction/features/bath-salts-drug-dangers

5. http://www.drugabuse.gov/publications/drugfacts/synthetic-cathinones-bath-salts

6. http://teens.drugabuse.gov/drug-facts/bath-salts

7. http://teens.drugabuse.gov/drug-facts/bath-salts

8. 9. http://www.drugabuse.gov/drugs-abuse/mdma-ecstasymolly

9. http://www.drugabuse.gov/publications/drugfacts/mdma-ecstasy-or-molly

10. http://teens.drugabuse.gov/drug-facts/mdma-ecstasy-or-molly

11. http://www.drugs.com/illicit/ghb.html

12. http://www.drugabuse.gov/publications/drugfacts/club-drugs-ghb-ketamine-rohypnol

13. http://www.drugfree.org/drug-guide/ghb/

14. http://www.drugabuse.gov/publications/drugfacts/khat

15. http://www.deadiversion.usdoj.gov/drug_chem_info/khat.pdf

16. http://www.dea.gov/pubs/pressrel/pr072606a.html

17. http://www.streetdrugs.org/html%20 les/Khat.html

18. http://www.drugs.com/illicit/krokodil.html

19. http://time.com/3398086/the-worlds-deadliest-drug-inside-a-krokodil-cookhouse/

20. http://www.drugs.com/illicit/rohypnol.html

21. http://www.drugfreeworld.org/drugfacts/prescription/rohypnol.html

22. http://www.drugabuse.gov/publications/drugfacts/club-drugs-ghb-ketamine-rohypnol

23. http://teens.drugabuse.gov/drug-facts/salvia

24. http://www.vice.com/read/why-is-salvia-so-uniquely-terrifying-1015

25. http://www.webmd.com/parenting/features/salvia-faq

26. http://www.drugabuse.gov/publications/drugfacts/salvia

27. 28. http://www.drugfree.org/drug-guide/k2-spice/

28. http://www.drugabuse.gov/publications/drugfacts/spice-synthetic-marijuana

29. http://www.rensco.com/pdfs/Health/SynMar/Product%20Names%20of%20Synthetic%20Marijuana.pdf

About the Author

Reid Lofgran has practiced as a family physician for over 16 years in rural Idaho. He is also the medical director of the Walker Center, a 28-day residential drug and alcohol treatment facility. Additionally, he provides office-based addiction treatment. After getting a bachelor's degree in Zoology at Brigham Young University Reid attended Kirksville College of Osteopathic Medicine in Kirksville Missouri, followed by additional training in Trenton, Michigan. Reid is happily married, with six children, a daughter-in-law, and 2 grandchildren. He enjoys writing, art, music, travel, being in the outdoors, and most of all, being with family. Reid enjoys serving in the church, having served many years in scouting, as young men's president, as bishop, and as high priest group leader. Reid enjoys speaking to youth and adults about preventing and treating addiction. www.reidlofgran.com

CPSIA information can be obtained
at www.ICGtesting.com
Printed in the USA
LVOW06s0922291217
561198LV00007B/18/P

9 780999 343005